A Neurobiologic View of Speech Production and the Dysarthrias

A Neurobiologic View of Speech Production and the Dysarthrias

Ronald Netsell, Ph.D.
Boys Town National Institute for
Communication Disorders in Children

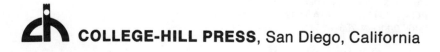 **COLLEGE-HILL PRESS**, San Diego, California

College-Hill Press, Inc.
4284 41st Street
San Diego, CA 92105

Library of Congress Cataloging-in Publication Data

Netsell, Ronald.
    A neurobiologic view of speech production and the
dysarthrias.

    Includes bibliographies and index.
    1. Articulation disorders. 2. Speech–Physiological
aspects.   I. Title.   [DNLM: 1. Nervous System Diseases
—Complications.   2. Speech—physiology.   3. Speech
Disorders—physiopathology.   WL 340 N471n]
RC424.7.N47   616.85'52   85-17404
ISBN 0-88744-206-4

Printed in United States of America

CONTENTS

Foreword   by Leonard L. LaPointe vii

Chapter 1.   The Acquisition of Speech Motor Control:
             A Perspective with Directions for Research 1

Chapter 2.   Speech Motor Control and
             Selected Neurologic Disorders 33

Chapter 3.   A Neurobiologic View of the Dysarthrias 53

Chapter 4.   Speech Motor Control:
             Theoretical Issues with Clinical Impact 89

Chapter 5.   Physiologic Studies of Dysarthria
             and Their Relevance to Treatment 105

Chapter 6.   Treating the Dysarthrias 123
             Ronald Netsell and John Rosenbek

Author Index 153

Subject Index 159

FOREWORD

Prior to the 1970s the realm of speech motor control and neurologic impairment of speech was practically *terra incognita* in the world of human communication. No one suggested that those who ventured into those relatively uncharted mists would fall off the edge of the earth, but risk-takers were few. Through the ages, passing nods were afforded the dysarthrias, but a systematic science was excruciatingly slow to develop, and application of the meager knowledge that had evolved was infrequent. Even within the infant discipline of speech-language pathology, focus on motor speech problems has been a recent development, except for some attention to "cerebral-palsied speech." Much has changed in the last 20 years. As one researcher who was instrumental in giving impetus to clinical research on motor speech processes recently stated, "Dysarthria appears to have come into its own" (Darley, 1983, p. xiii).

Cursory allusions, vague hints, and occasional references have given way to an abundance of books, chapters, reviews, and a growing empirical data base that has sprung from purposeful efforts in both laboratory and clinic. Traditionally, people afflicted with speech-language disorders had been sent home, given a gloomy prognosis, or tentatively treated as if the clinicians were walking on eggs. Now at least some are afforded behavioral and prosthetic intervention options that serve genuinely to alter the quality of their lives.

A more fundamental issue, advancement of what we know about the mechanisms of speech motor control in both normal and neurologically compromised people, has been appropriately intertwined with attention to management of the dysarthrias. For years measurement and appreciation of speech movements was rudimentary at best and awaited the boost provided by technological advances of the 1960s and 1970s.

Research on speech motor control and on neuromotor speech impairment has been carried out in only a handful of clinics and laboratories across the world, several of them clustered in the midwestern United States. What has emerged has been a satisfying direction as to how we conceptualize speech production in both its normal and aberrant state. What has begun to crystallize is the concept of a physiologic approach or a neurobiologic view of motor speech behavior. Attention to speech motor control in both the normal and the pathologic state has proved fruitful and beneficial to both states. Study of motor speech impairment has helped us gain a measure of understanding of the normal speech production process, and study of nonimpaired speech has led to applications in the clinic.

A principal proponent and formulator of this neurobiologic view of motor speech production has been Ronald Netsell. His work has been well recognized for nearly 20 years and is firmly grounded on an empirical, data-based research tradition, with an eye on application.

The careful scholar will notice that as early as 1967 Netsell was acknowledged in a landmark article by J. C. Hardy entitled "Suggestions for physiologic research in dysarthria," published in the then new journal of neurobehavior, *Cortex*. "Special recognition is due to Ronald W. Netsell, M.A., Research Assistant, for his work on cinefluorography with dysarthric subjects" (Hardy, 1967, p. 154). One of Hardy's stated purposes of this article was to ". . . stimulate research and thinking regarding neuromuscular pathologies of the speech producing mechanisms" (p. 129), and Netsell's subsequent efforts contributed to the fulfillment of that purpose.

Since those early days in Iowa, Netsell has labored in the Speech Motor Control Laboratories at the University of Wisconsin, Madison, and the Human Communications Laboratories of the Boys Town National Institute. He now has a firm base of empirical research, and much of his most recent writing has focused on sythesizing, drawing together, reviewing, postulating, and tidying-up what we know about speech production. His reviews are always incisive and instructive. As Barnett has commented, "These days top-flight, productive, competitive scientists who write many review chapters are like the road agents of yesteryear who were glorified in tale and song. [They must approach the task] with style and judgment, wearing a greased holster and drawing in a slick fashion" (Barnett, 1983, p. 341).

This book is a collection of some of Netsell's work in the 1980s, gathered from widely scattered sources compiled and published in a single book. As such it serves to preserve and draw together a cohesive chunk of contemporary knowledge about neuromotor speech production.

Netsell was not easy to convince that this collection of his work should be assembled and published. Despite his reservations, Netsell has been persuaded that this collection deserves to be shared and, in fact, contributes to the advancement of the science.

The increasingly interdisciplinary character of the study of human goal-directed movement assures that members of many disciplines could benefit from this book. Students and researchers in psychology, kinesiology, and neurophysiology who are interested in motor control, particularly as reflected in the act of speech production, will be rewarded by this work.

Perhaps more so than others, students, clinicians, and researchers in speech-language pathology will find relevant information here. These writings reflect a period of significant advancement in our understanding of motor speech issues, and Netsell's work, as much as anyone's, represents a bridge between the laboratory and the clinic. More of these bridges should be built, and they need to be heavily traveled. Clinical decisions related to the management of motor speech impairment are becoming more firmly grounded in empiricism, and the chapters of this book strongly illuminate that trend. Understanding the veiled and complicated mechanisms of motor speech production is a necessary and laudable objective, but, as Darley suggested, "... the most important things we can know about the dysarthrias are how to reduce them and help flesh-and-blood patients cope with them" (Darley, 1983, p. xv).

In these chapters the reader will find contrasts between adult models and acquisition, minima of normal range and velocity of speech movements, postulates on the existence of microanatomy for speech movements, descriptions of specific disorders of muscle forcing functions, descriptions of speech correlates to physiologic aberration for several neuropathologies, and (in collaboration with John C. Rosenbek, a clinician who sets standards to be emulated) specific principles and suggestions to guide individualized treatment of motor speech impairment. A book that covers these important issues with the caution and the thought exhibited by Netsell is worth its salt, worth its lime, and worth its oyster.

The precious and fragile nature of human speech has been rhapsodized and lamented in prose for centuries. The limitations and unrealized potential of communication, particularly after the nervous system has been impaired, is reflected in the following observation:

> Human speech is like a cracked kettle on which we tap crude rhythms for bears to dance to, while we long to make music that will melt the stars.
> (Flaubert, 1857)

When the nervous system is cracked the rhythms of speech can be cruder, but thanks to the efforts of clinical scientists such as Netsell, our appreciation and understanding of speech motor control is evolving at a satisfying rate. This book is testament to a significant period in that advancement and also assures continuity by indicating directions for future graduate assistants.

Leonard L. LaPointe
Arizona State University

REFERENCES

Barnett, R.J. (1983). Review of *Modern cell biology. The Yale Journal of Biology and Medicine, 56*, 341.

Darley, F.L. (1983). Foreword. In W. Berry (Ed.), *Clinical dysarthria*. San Diego: College Hill Press.

Flaubert, G. (1957). *Madame Bovary* (F. Steegmuller, Trans.). New York: Random House. (Original work published 1857).

Hardy, J.C. (1967). Suggestions for physiologic research in dysarthria. *Cortex, 3*, 128-156.

Chapter 1

The Acquisition of Speech Motor Control: A Perspective with Directions for Research

The content of this chapter will focus on *speech* production as a *motor control system*, hence the term "speech motor control" in the title. The term "acquisition" is used to designate speech production as a *motor skill*. This speech motor skill undergoes a long period of acquisition (perhaps to early adolescence), has several developmental prerequisites (especially neuro-anatomic-physiologic and musculoskeletal), and is paralleled as a motor skill perhaps only by the unusual person who plays the piano entirely "by ear."

Almost all the declarative statements made in this chapter should be stated as hypotheses. However, as a convenience, the hypothetical form will be avoided for the most part. As a neophyte on the subject matter of this conference, perhaps I can be allowed to ask some of the old questions again that most of you have dealt with for years. In return, I might provide some information on speech motor control that will enhance the interpretation of existing data, condition somewhat the collection of new data, and provide the theory and model builders in language development with anatomic and physiologic hypotheses to account for much of the speech behavior seen in infancy and early childhood.

In reviewing several theories of phonologic development, Ferguson

Reprinted by permission of the publisher from *Language behavior in infancy and early childhood*, R. Stark (Ed.), pp. 127-156. Copyright 1981 by Elsevier Science Publishing Co., Inc., New York.

and Garnica (1975) suggest that a more cohesive and unifying theory probably could be pieced together from parts of the existing ones. More important, these authors state that

> the development of more satisfying theories of children's acquisition of phonology will not come from elaborate speculation, no matter how sophisticated linguistically, nor from large-scale data collection without reference to particular problems, but from principled investigations focused on specific hypotheses and questions of fact.
> (p. 176)

A corollary thesis of the present chapter is that these developmental theories would be strongly served by a solid base of *descriptive physiologic data* that underlies the speech acoustic patterns of the infant and young child. With an eye toward stimulating research in this area, the remainder of this chapter will focus on (1) understanding *adult speech motor control* in relation to *speech acquisition*; (2) a review of *neural maturation and motor control processes* believed to operate in the prenatal and two-year postnatal periods; and (3) speculations regarding *neural origins of speech movement*; it will also (4) introduce the concept of *speech motor age*; and (5) form *hypotheses* about the *acquisition of speech motor control* that are both testable and requisite to a more complete theory of language development.

ADULT MODELS AND SPEECH ACQUISITION

The physical act of speaking can be viewed as a series of transformations beginning with a set of neural effector commands that control more than 100 muscle contractions. These muscle contractions move the various peripheral structures depicted in Figure 1–1. The movements of these structures (bones, cartilages and muscles), in turn, generate the time-continuous acoustic waveform that we perceive as speech. The primary interest of speech motor control research is to characterize the muscle forces and structure movements in terms that ultimately allow inferences about the nature of the underlying neural control mechanisms. To both the casual and long-term observer of these procedures, these are very difficult problems to solve. Figure 1–1 shows the representation of the peripheral speech mechanism as a set of ten functional components.* The movements of these semi-independent parts act to generate air pressure and air flows. The points of aerodynamic measurement, also shown in Figure 1–1, become valuable indices of the speech movements as well as partial sources

---

*A *functional component* is defined as a structure, or set of structures, used to generate or valve the speech air stream.

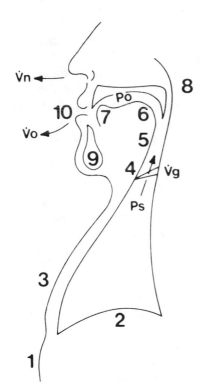

STRUCTURES

1 - abdominal muscles
2 - diaphragm
3 - ribcage
4 - larynx
5 - tongue/pharynx
6 - posterior tongue
7 - anterior tongue
8 - velopharynx
9 - jaw
10- lips

AERODYNAMICS

Ps - subglottal air pressure
Po - intraoral air pressure
Vg - glottal air flow
Vo - oral air flow
Vn - nasal air flow

Figure 1-1. A drawing of the vocal tract that shows functional components and aerodynamic variables involved in speech production.

for the generation of the speech acoustics. Together with the actual component part movements, the aerodynamic and acoustic-phonetic information probably holds the greatest promise for describing the acquisition of speech control. Undoubtedly, the age and cooperation of the particular subject will condition which types of measurement are feasible. Ideally, of course, measurements would be taken simultaneously from all levels of the speech production process.

Adult Speech Motor Control

This section is designed to acquaint the naive reader with certain properties and capabilities of the adult speech motor control system. The adult system is of interest when considering skill acquisition because it represents the end point of the developmental continuum and, as such, reflects the elegance to which the developing system aspires and can be compared. All the data on adult speech motor control are far from being in. The "hard facts" about the system properties and function are really very few. The greatest range of movement in the system is seen for the lips, tongue, and jaw, and this is about 1 to 1.5 cm. Typical velocities of movement for these structures are around 10–15 cm/s, with maximum speeds approaching 25 cm/s. The maximum rate of syllable repetition for the adult speaker is around 6 per second. For example, in trying to say *pa pa pa pa* at a rate faster than about 6 cm/s, most adults will begin to fuse the lip and laryngeal movements together such that the voiceless *p* consonant becomes voiced. The physical limitation appears to be the rate at which the vocal folds can be adducted and abducted across the outgoing air stream. The laryngeal muscles have one of the few clearly reciprocal muscle arrangements in the speech mechanism; this is the muscle system used to rapidly position the folds in and out of the air stream for contrasts such as voiced-voiceless consonants. In conversational speech, these in-and-out motions of the folds to the midline are accomplished in about 75 to 100 ms. In effect, then, certain laryngeal muscles are behaving as an articulator in the same way as do the lips, tongue, and velopharynx. This point is emphasized here because many earlier phonologic accounts emphasized the larynx as a sound source for voicing and a frequency generator for pitch. When viewed also as an articulation, the coordinative role of the vocal folds with the lips, tongue, and other structures becomes critical, as reflected in the voice onset time (VOT) measure. Interestingly, the VOT does not reach adult-like precision until around age 11 (Kent, 1976). However, the VOT does not represent the time minima of coordination between two articulators in the adult system. For example, for various *sp* consonant strings the tongue-alveolus constriction for the *s* is never released prior to the complete lip closure for *p* and never delays more than 10 ms in releasing after the bilabial lip seal has been completed (Kent and Moll, 1975). Thus, the adult speech system has time minima for such coordinations as fine as 10 ms.

Another intriguing feature of the adult speech motor system is the subconscious manner with which speech movements are made. If normal adults hold rigid pieces between their teeth and produce the vowel *i*, their tongues will assume almost identical positions in the high-front regions of the oral cavity and they will produce nearly identical acoustic-perceptual *i* vowels without any conscious repositioning of the tongue. The summary of preliminary data from one such experiment is shown in Figure 1–2 (from Netsell, Kent, and Abbs, 1978). The left side of the figure shows superimpositions of tongue shapes for three speakers; solid lines are with the jaw free to move and dashed lines are with the upper and lower incisors separated by a 16 mm spacer. The tongue shapes on the right side of Figure 1–2 are referenced to the mandible and show the extent to which each subject subconsciously repositioned the tongue to produce the vowel *i* when the jaw was in a fixed position. An even more striking feature of this subconscious motor control of speech is shown in Figure 1–3. The same three

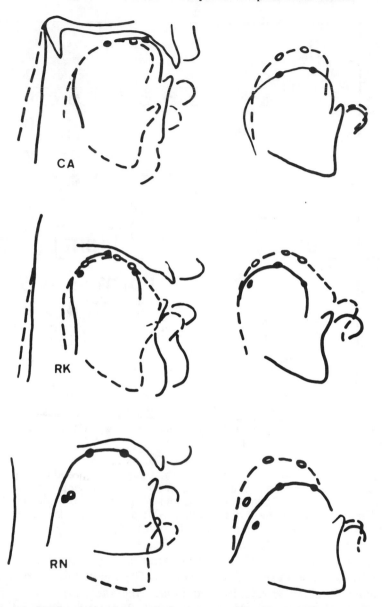

Figure 1–2. Midsagittal line drawings of the upper airway for *i* vowel productions by three adult speakers. *Left side:* Superimpositions of lips, tongue, and pharynx when the jaw was free to move (solid lines) and held in a fixed position (dashed lines). *Right side:* Superimpositions of tongue shapes referenced to the jaw which shows the extent of adjustment made with the tongue to achieve the similar tongue positions on the left. From Netsell, R., Kent, R., and Abbs, J. (1978).

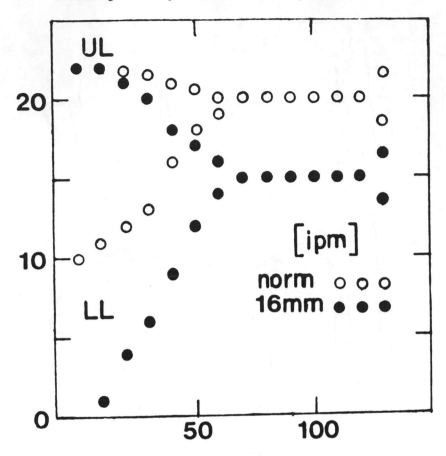

Figure 1–3. Time-motion displays for the upper lip (UL) and lower lip (LL) resulting from production of the *ea* and *m* sounds in the sentence "You h*eap my* hay high happy." Open circles: Lip movement with jaw participating. Filled circles: Lip movement with the jaw in a fixed position (see text for details). From Netsell, R., Kent, R., and Abbs, J. (1978).

subjects repeated the sentence "you heap my hay high happy" with the jaw free to vary and in three fixed positions. The use of this more natural language production revealed additional remarkable capabilities of the adult speech motor control system. Figure 1–3 contrasts upper and lower lip movements, with and without the jaw fixed, for the "heap my" segments of the test sentence. With the upper and lower incisors separated by the 16 mm spacer, the lips moved a greater distance to make the lip closure for *p*. Interestingly, they moved this distance at a greater velocity (especially the lower lip) such that the movement of lip closure was achieved in the same time interval as the control (jaw free) condition. The point of lip contact was made 5 mm lower for the jaw fixed condition. Moreover, the lip seal for the *mp* segments was maintained for the same period of time in both speaking conditions. As in the isolated vowel productions depicted in Figure 1–2, none of the subjects reported any awareness of these temporal and spatial adjustments recorded in the jaw fixed conditions. Further examination of these data, which is now under way, should reveal particular temporal-spatial minima in the jaw fixed conditions (i.e., points in time that the controller may deem most necessary to bring the vocal tract into a particular shape to yield the necessary acoustic equivalents of the jaw free, or normal speech conditions). As such, these temporal-spatial minima may reflect something about the motor goals of the neural control system. Clearly, it would be of considerable interest to learn when children develop this level of subconscious control of their speech motor output. Rutherford (1967) and Hardy (1970), among others, have speculated that children place their emerging speech movements under a rather direct afferent monitoring system, in which auditory and movement cues are used to help refine the positional and temporal control of the developing speech movements. At some unknown time, these more overt monitoring systems fade into a background where the child no longer uses them. Whether or not the children really use afferent cues in a conscious or subconscious manner also is not known. If they do, it is not at all clear when they begin to produce speech unconsciously, as we adults too often do.

Speech Acquisition

The relationships described earlier that may be used in the acquisition of speech are diagrammed in Figure 1–4. It is hypothesized that the normal child learns to talk by listening, watching, and imitating an external model

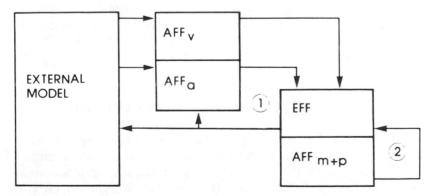

Figure 1-4. A block diagram of elements hypothesized to function in the acquisition of speech motor control (see text for details).

(e.g., a parent, caregiver or another child). The model provides both auditory and visual afferent cues (AFFa and AFFv), which the child attempts to imitate with his or her own movements and vocalizations (shown as EFF, efferent). This EFF has two important consequences.

First, it generates the auditory patterns that return to the ears of the model and to the child himself. The latter auditory feedback closes the important motor-auditory loop as in 1 in Figure 1–4. Second, EFF creates feedback associated with the speech movements and postures (AFFm+p) that the child pairs with his own auditory patterns. In essence, he hears and "feels" his speech movements as they are being developed. This tight sensorimotor-auditory coupling presumably is the key to his refinement of output (EFF) to approximate the external model. By this process, the child eventually develops internal representation in his nervous system of these sensorimotor-auditory patterns.

Speech as a Motor Control System

We seem no closer today than we were ten years ago to understanding or even conceptualizing the nature of speech as a motor control system (Kent and Minifie, 1977; Lindblom, Lubker, and Gay, 1979; MacNeilage and Ladefoged, 1976). Whether the system is under open or closed loop control, or both, or whether it is preprogrammed and playing out a motor tape while oblivious to its senses remains a matter of essential conjecture. Many researchers seem stymied as to the critical experiments to perform, but the multidisciplinary research at the Speech Motor Control Laboratories at the University of Wisconsin holds considerable promise (Abbs, 1979, personal communication; Abbs, Muller, Hassul, and Netsell, 1977). Researchers of speech motor acquisition should watch closely the outcome of the above-mentioned adult experiments for cues to useful paradigms. A similar watchful eye should be kept on the "shadowing paradigms" at the Louisiana State University Medical Center (Porter, 1978; Porter and Castellanos, 1980; Porter and Lubker, 1980).

NEURAL MATURATION AND MOTOR CONTROL

The temporal courses and eventual attainment of adult speech motor control seem most dependent on the individual's nervous system maturation. The study of neural maturation is by no means a straightforward matter, and Yakovlev's distinctions (1962) between *development, growth,* and *maturation* will be used here in forming a working definition of *neural maturation.*

Definitions and Perspectives

Yakovlev (1962) depicted growth and maturation as subordinate and additive to his concept of development:

> The development of the nervous system follows a sequence of morphological events which reflect and correlate with the changes in the internal state, outward form and dynamic relations of the organism to the environment. All these changes are subsumed in the conceptions of growth and maturation of the biological action systems. The conception of *maturation*, however, has a broader connotation of an exponential process of the progressive organization of functions and of their morphological substrata which go on through the life span of the individual. . . . (p. 3, italics added)

Yakovlev's definition of *neural maturation* contains both morphologic and functional components (i.e., a process of "progressive organization of functions and their morphological substrata"). This definition fits well with the concept of "systemogenesis" (Anokhin, 1964). Anokhin hypothesized that motor behavior was governed by a number of functional systems within the nervous system. A functional system was made up of a group of nervous system structures that developed an "action-system specificity." For example, the neuroanatomy and neurophysiology subserving swallowing would be one such functional system and that subserving speech production would be a second functional system. Given this scheme, swallowing and speech could share certain neuroanatomic structures while maintaining separate neural functional systems. These systems are said to develop on different schedules, according to the needs of the organism. Therefore, the functional system for swallowing is developed *in utero* so that it can be ready for use at birth. The functional system for speech motor control, on the other hand, is not present at birth. Indeed, as will be indicated in more detail later, it appears the neural functional system for speech is not in place until near the end of the second year of life.

Criteria for Neural and Motor Maturation

The five criteria used here in a discussion of neural maturation are myelination, axonal-dendritic growth, nerve cell proliferation, synaptogenesis, and changes in the electroencephalogram (EEG). These criteria are emphasized because of their frequent appearance in the speech and language literature. Myelination is used with the caution that many neurons may be quite functional in a given system without a myelin sheath. The more judicious use of the myelin criterion is to regard *full* myelination of a given set of neurons as evidence of full, or nearly complete, maturation of that part of a functional system. The two criteria used in this chapter to reflect motor maturation are status of the primitive reflexes (after Capute, Accardo, Vining, Rubenstein, and Harryman, 1978) and movements associated with vegetation (sucking, swallowing, chewing, etc.), sound production (crying, vocalization, verbalization, etc.), and walking.

"Critical" and "Sensitive" Periods

Clearly, embryogenesis and other fetal developments represent critical periods in the infant's maturation. As Ferry, Culbertson, Fitzgibbons, and Netzky (1979) point out,

> The concept of various critical periods in neurologic development has been proposed to indicate finite items in which specific events must occur to provide the substrate for subsequent developmental achievements. This "now-or-never" hypothesis is based upon imprinting studies in animals and psychologic studies of sensorimotor development leading to cognitive skills in children.
>
> More recently, however, the concept has been challenged. Wolff, in 1970, suggested that child behavior depends upon the complex interaction of many biologic and environmental factors. The concept of "sensitive" periods has been proposed as an alternative, referring to periods when a child may learn particular skills more easily than others.
>
> Based on the early precocity of brain development and the highly complex interaction between neurogenesis, synaptogenesis, and myelination as described, all phases of early brain development are critical. The most important (if not critical) period of neurologic development is the first 10 weeks of intrauterine life, when the anatomic, physiologic, and biochemical substrates of future developmental progress are being formed. (p. 15)

One of the theses to be developed in this chapter is that the acquisition of speech motor control is a continuous but nonlinear process. Sensitive periods of nonlinearity occur when certain neural, musculoskeletal, environmental, and cognitive changes combine (or "get together") in the individual organism. The points in time at which a particular number of these factors combine can result in jumps in performance that appear incremental, if not placed on a conceptually broader map of sensorimotor and cognitive development.

Because the environmental impact upon the natural course of neural and motor maturation probably will eternally blur the "innate versus acquired" distinction, we are basically left with the construction of milestone maps that chart the age ranges at which particular neuroanatomic, sensory, motor, and cognitive functions presumably are available. The following paragraphs will draw attention to particular periods of change in motor control in general (and speech motor control in particular) and corresponding changes in the maturation of the nervous system. Obviously no cause-effect relationship can be drawn from the temporal coincidence of reported motor control and neural maturation changes. Nevertheless, the correspondence of these neural and musculoskeletal developments will lead to a number of hypotheses that are in need of investigation.

PRENATAL PERIOD

Neuronal Maturation. In the period of 4 to 9 fetal months, several basic neural structures apparently undergo considerable or nearly complete myelination including the lower motoneurons, prethalamic auditory pathways, the pre- and postthalamic exteroceptive and proprioceptive routes, and portions of the inferior cerebellar peduncle (Fig. 1–5).* Parenthetically, it should be noted that the postthalamic auditory pathways do not fully myelinate until around the fourth or fifth year!

Motor Control. The fetus during this time is developing a number of movement routines, some of which will be called into action as he moves at birth from the medium of water to air. Anokhin (1964) points out that the neural functional systems to support survival at birth (namely, breathing, sucking, and swallowing) are developed and fully practiced at this period. Indeed, at birth, the facial nerve connections to the lips are complete while those to other muscles of facial expression are not. The most cited studies of fetal movements are those of Hooker and Humphrey (see review in Humphrey, 1971) in which responses of aborted fetuses to tactile stimuli were documented with motion picture film. Evoked fetal movements ranged from total body reactions to orofacial responses, including sucking, swallowing, gagging, and jaw extension, among others. In this stimulus-response paradigm, even independence of lip and jaw movement was reported for the 25-week-old fetus. Although the young aborted fetus often initiates breathing, implying sufficient neural innervation of the diaphragm, it is estimated that full innervation of the respiratory system is not complete until approximately 8 months after birth (Bouhuys, 1971).

---

*Figure 1–5 is a reproduction of Lecours's (1975) "myelogenetic" chart (taken in part from Yakovlev and Lecours, 1967). Mindful of the caution given earlier, it is assumed that the extent of myelination of the various nervous system regions is a reasonable first approximation of their functional maturation. Concurrent and subsequent accounts provide important details on other maturational criteria, but they do not result in major revisions of the Yakovlev-Lecours myelin map. (Jacobson, 1975; Lecours, 1975; Milner 1976; Scheibel and Scheibel, 1976; Sloan, 1967; Whitaker, 1976). Myelination functions are shown for 10 nervous system regions believed to play some role in the acquisition of speech motor control. The functions span the time period from the 4-month-old fetus through 15 postnatal years. Related developments are shown for certain speech and language variables (rows A–F in Figure 1–5).

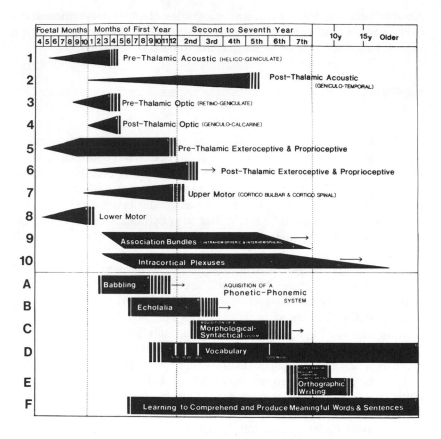

Figure 1-5. Table of myelination in selected portions of the nervous system (rows 1-10) and related development of certain speech and language variables (rows A-F). Reprinted from Lecours, A. (1975). Myelogenetic correlates of the development of speech and language. In E. Lenneberg and E. Lenneberg (Eds.), *Foundations of language development. A multidisciplinary approach*, (Vol. 1, pp. 121-136). New York: Academic Press. Reprinted with permission.

THE NEONATE (BIRTH TO 3 MONTHS)

Neural Maturation. According to the myelination charts, the major neural connections being formed and nearly completed in this period are the pre- and postthalamic optic tracts. An important event of myelination with respect to sensorimotor control that begins at or near birth involves the upper motoneuron (corticospinal and corticobulbar) tracts and postthalamic auditory and somatosensory pathways. First evidences of myelination are also reported in this period for the middle cerebellar peduncle, corpus striatum, and frontopontine pathway. The inner cell layers of cerebral cortex (especially the primary motor and sensory areas) are fairly well developed in this period, suggesting that some of the observed movement patterns of the newborn are utilizing the cortical levels (Milner, 1976). However, the secondary and association areas are regarded as nonfunctional at this point, as evidenced in both axonal-dendritic connections and EEG activity (Milner, 1976; Woodruff, 1978). For the most part, primitive reflexes are obligatory in this period, and the general assumption is that they remain so until the cortical mechanisms begin to inhibit them at about three months (Capute et al., 1978). The consensus seems to be that subcortical neural mechanisms dominate in this period. Woodruff's statement (1978) is representative of this view:

> The parallels between human and monkey development and the similar concordance between EEG alpha onset and the disappearance of primitive reflexes in both species provide evidence that normal infants are functionally subcortical organisms (Lindsley and Wicks, 1974). These authors find additional evidence for subcortical dominance in neonates in the developmental parallels between normal infants and anencephalic monsters in the first 2 months of life. Born without a cerebral cortex, anencephalic monsters do not survive more than 2 months, but while they live they show reflex development similar to the patterns of normal human infants of the same age. (p. 125)

Motor Control. Corresponding to its neuroanatomic status, the visual motor system of the newborn is quite highly developed. Oculomotor control for object following and object and person recognition (implying higher levels of function) is seen within the first few weeks following birth (Wolff, 1969). The most notable motor act of the newborn for the listener is crying. The cry has its own developmental course (Bosma, Truby, and Lind, 1965; Stark and Nathanson, 1973; Wolff, 1969). It is debatable that the respiratory-laryngeal mechanics, muscle forces, and aerodynamics developed in crying are prerequisites or corequisites to the development of respiratory-laryngeal controls used for speaking* (see Moyers, 1971). The forceful cries associated with pain or other distress can be generated with subglottal air pressures in excess of 60 cm H_2O (where values of 5 to 10 cm H_2O are used for child and adult speech) and both the rib cage and abdominal muscles contract vigorously (Bosma et al., 1965; Hixon, 1979, personal communication). Acoustic-physiologic studies of infant vocalizations in "nondistress" modes probably are considerably closer to the respiratory-laryngeal controls used for speech development (Langlois and Baken, 1976; Wilder and Baken, 1974, 1978). It is not surprising that the

---

*This potentially provoking statement is discussed in a later section dealing with the neurogenics of speech production and vegetative movements (sucking, swallowing, chewing, etc.).

vocalizations toward the end of this first 90 days of life are largely vocalic, nasalized, and of short duration (Nakazima, 1975; Oller, 1978; Wolff, 1969). Preliminary observations suggest the respiratory contributions to these vocalizations are made entirely in the expiratory phase of tidal breathing and without opposition of rib cage and abdominal movements (Baken, 1979, personal communication; Hixon, 1979, personal communication).

All sound productions of the infant indicate a rather simple function for the larynx. In terms of upper airway movements, (1) there is no indication the velopharynx is alternately opening and closing for speech, (2) the tongue and jaw move as a single piece to effect velar-like stops (with the infant reclining or on his back) or apicals (e.g., *da-da-da* or *na-na-na*), (3) lip-jaw independence seldom is seen for front-of-the-mouth speech movements in this period. This lack of tongue or lip independence from jaw movements during speech-like vocalizations of this period stands in contrast to lip-jaw independence in smiling (Wolff, 1969) or tongue-lip responses independent of jaw movement in response to tactile stimuli (Weiffenbach and Thach, 1973).

In summary, the neonate appears as a rather unsophisticated sound generator (by adult standards) who may occasionally surprise himself and his other listeners with "speech" by simply opening and closing his mouth while phonating.

THE BABBLER (3 TO 12 MONTHS)

As is suggested later from the review of neural and motor correlates, 3 to 12 months may be the single most *sensitive postnatal period* with respect to the eventual acquisition of *normal speech motor control.** Delays or other abnormalities that appear or remain in this period would seem to have extremely serious consequences in terms of building in the fundamental speech movement routines that are later refined in the overall coordination of the speech mechanism. In addition, it is a period of rather dramatic changes in the musculoskeletal system (Kent, 1981). As a consequence, the morphologic and functional plasticity of the maturing nervous system is put to test in this early period and neurologic abnormalities detected here would seem to have high clinical value. Speech motor control descriptions of individual functional components (see Figure 1–1) and their developing coordination may prove to be a relatively sensitive index of neuromotor maturation and, as such, provide diagnostic and prognostic additions to the clinical neurologic examination.

*See earlier distinction between "sensitive" and "critical" periods on page 10.

Neural Maturation. Major developments occur here in pyramidal tract (corticospinal and corticobulbar) myelination as well as postthalamic somatosensory pathways. The major development in "hard wiring" of the middle cerebellar peduncle is formed in this period, and the input-output at this level of the cerebellum is generally regarded as the key neural component for cerebellar function in speech motor control. In addition, the beginnings and completion of corpus striatum myelination occur in this nine-month period (see Yakovlev and Lecours, 1967), and this seems a reasonable neuroanatomic correlate for the postural and movement developments that are outlined later. Taken together, these motor corticofugal-striatal-cerebellar-thalamic-sensorimotor cortical connections are forming a network of loops or circuits that are most strongly implicated in more recent theories of fine motor control (see Desmedt, 1978, for review). Also of major importance to the development of speech motor control is the considerable myelination seen in the postthalamic auditory projections. Assuming the child is forming critical "auditory-motor linkages" at this time (see Ladefoged, DeClerk, Lindau, and Papcun, 1972; MacNeilage and Ladefoged, 1976), the already described neuroanatomic developments of the motor, somatosensory, and auditory systems are quite timely.

As the primitive reflex patterns remit, presumably due to cortical inhibition, clear organization in EEG activity appears (Milner, 1976; Woodruff, 1978). Using the visual system development in illustration, Bronson (quoted by Woodruff) suggests that a secondary, subcortical, and phylogenetically older visual system regulates visual behavior in the first three months and is superseded by a cortically controlled system thereafter.

> In a recent review of the literature on neonatal visual behavior, Bronson (1974) argued that newborns rely on a phylogenetically older "subcortical" "second visual system" in the first months of life, and it is only in the third month that the newer (cortical) "primary visual system" dominates. Bronson (1974) contended that rather than conceiving postnatal changes in visual behavior as indicative of general improvement in the efficiency of the total system, changes in visual behavior in infancy can be interpreted in terms of underlying neural changes corresponding to the progressive development of increasingly sophisticated neural networks. Specifically, the progression involves first a subcortical system located in the superior colliculus and pulvinar, which is involved in processing stimulation falling on the more peripheral areas of the retina. This system functions to transmit information about direction of salient peripherally located stimuli and is not capable of analyzing patterns. As development progresses, another system takes precedence. This is the primary visual system, the geniculostriate system involving foveal vision and pattern detection.
>
> (p. 125–126 in Woodruff, 1978)

In review of work by Hecox (1975), Woodruff (1978) points to parallels in development for the visual and auditory evoked potentials, VER and AER, respectively:

> Hecox presented evidence that both peripheral and central mechanisms are responsible for higher thresholds to auditory stimuli in infancy. The neurophysiological data indicated that the human infant is more sensitive to auditory stimuli at a brainstem level than had been indicated by the behavioral data. The more rostral the response is processed in the auditory system, the higher the threshold. Thus, Hecox presented new electrophysiological evidence that in the auditory system, brainstem or subcortical mechanisms mature earlier than cortical mechanisms. This provides evidence for parallel developmental patterns in auditory and visual systems and suggests that neonates operate at subcortical levels early in life. (p. 144)

Comparisons of waveform shape and peak delays for the VER, AER, and SER (somatosensory evoked response) in the infant and child would seem to hold considerable promise developing sensory maturation profiles.

Motor Control. There may be a transition between the periods of the neonate and babbler that marks the onset of emergence for movement subroutines that will eventually form the efferent-afferent (auditory-movement-somatosensory feedback) substrata of adult speech motor control. We'll call this period that of the *ya*bbler in recognition of the *yeah* sound the infant can produce by simply raising and lowering the jaw fast enough to blend the /i/ and /ae/ vowels together. The early period of the babbler also marks the infant's initial struggle with gravity in terms of probable effects on speech production. In beginning to speak while sitting up or semireclining, the 3 month old infant almost spontaneously assumes adult-like usage of rib cage and abdominal movements (Hixon, 1979, personal communication). The partitions of lung volume and inspiratory-expiratory ratios used in speaking at 7 months are essentially adult-like (Baken, 1979, personal communication). Baken also reports the adult-like respiratory patterns for speech are formed shortly after the child assumes the vertical alignments of the head, neck, and torso. Gravity effects also are posited to affect mandibular function, downward-forward growth of the mandible is more rapid than other craniofacial expansions (Moyers, 1971), the larynx moves markedly downward (around 4 to 6 months) as the mandible-hyoid-laryngeal suspension system develops, and the upper airway assumes more adult-like dimensions (Kent, 1981). The immature swallow pattern of the infant (with tongue fronting and single piece, plunger-like action of the jaw and lips) is giving way to a more mature swallow with tongue retraction and more independence of lip and jaw movement. The appearance of front teeth increases tongue retraction and lip, tongue, and jaw movements become more independent in the early stages of chew ing (Fletcher, 1971; Moyers, 1971). No study was found in the literature that examined the correspondence of orofacial movements developed in feeding (and especially chewing) and the emergence of speech movement. A motion picture study of infant feeding and speech movements is in progress (Morris, 1979, personal communication).

Against this background of neural maturation, musculoskeletal growth, and vegetative orofacial development is the emergence of movements in the same peripheral structures for the motor control of speech.

In a later section of this chapter, the hypothesis is developed that the vegetative and speech movements emerge in parallel and are not sequentially dependent. Various accounts of the acoustic-phonetic sound pattern changes in this period give clues as to the increases in speech motor skill (Morris, 1980; Nakazima, 1975; Oller, 1978). Two to four syllables appear in a single expiration and the more typical shapes are consonant-vowel (CV), vowel-consonant (VC), and vowel-consonant-vowel (VCV). In terms of motor complexity, it should be noted that this requires only that the child start with the oral tract constricted and open it (CV), start with it open and close it (VC), or open-close-open (VCV). A parsimonious hypothesis is that through the *ya*bbling period the infant begins generating these basic syllable types by simply lowering and elevating the jaw while phonating. Somewhere between 3 and 9 months jaw independence from lower lip and tongue movements emerges for most normal children, as inferred from reports of consonant productions such as *r, s, z, th,* and *w.* A full range of vowels and diphthongs also is developed in this period, implicating shifts and shaping of the entire tongue body. The voiced-voiceless contrast is established routinely by 6 months and this suggests the adductor-abductor muscles of the larynx have at least the beginnings of reciprocal action. Finer gradations of voice fundamenal frequency for pitch variations in phrases of declaration and question indicate more precise control of muscle contraction (e.g., *cricothyroideus*) in a nonreciprocal situation. Finally, the appearance of nasal-nonnasal contrasts *m/b* and *n/d* in this period signals the probability that at least gross contractions of the *palatal levator* take place. It seems reasonable to predict from the adult physiology also that the nasal contrast would precede the voicing contrast developmentally because complete or nearly complete velopharyngeal closure accompanies the voiceless consonant productions.

THE TODDLER (12 TO 24 MONTHS)

Reference to other motor milestones shows that most 12 month olds are beginning to walk at about the time of their first words (Shirley, 1959). The practice of walking *or* talking seems sufficient to "tie up" all the available sensorimotor circuitry because the toddler seldom, if ever, undertakes both activities at once. As will be developed later, this period is marked by considerable practice and refinement of speech motor skills acquired in the previous period as well as the acquisition of more and more complex speech movement patterns.

Neural Maturation. A close look at Figure 1–5 reveals that full myelination of the postthalamic somesthetic pathways is not complete for most normal children until about 18 months, also a point at which most children walk unaided. From a speech motor perspective, this final "hard wiring" of the somatosensory pathway puts the child in touch with his cerebral cortex, and motor cortex in particular, such that the emerging speech movement patterns can be practiced using the full range of the fast acting cortical-cerebellar-somatosensory-thalamic-cortical loops.* Myelination of the postthalamic auditory pathways are continuing at a moderate rate. Considerable growth occurs in cerebral neocortex during the 12- to 24-month period, especially in the middle and anterior sections (Milner, 1976). Most of the layers of the cortex are vertically connected with respect to the neuraxis, and horizontal connections between association areas are just getting under way. Myelination of the cerebral commissures, which was initiated in the previous period, shows a rather marked growth in the second year, but does not near completion until about the end of the seventh year (see Milner, 1976; Yakovlev and Lecours, 1967). The rather sparse connections of the cortical association areas coupled with the myelination rate of the hemispheric connecting commissures may have been part of the rationale for Gazzaniga's hypothesis that infants are functionally "split-brained" with good interhemispheric function not being realized until age 2 to 3 years (Gazzaniga, 1970).

Motor Control. The emergence of words in this period coincides nicely with (1) the completion of "hard wiring" in the major sensorimotor pathways believed to operate in speech motor control, and (2) a period of stabilization in musculoskeletal growth. In puzzling over how the child might generate speech movement patterns for new words, the inescapable question arises as to what size of "movement units" are being developed and practiced.

---

*This so-called "hard wiring" refers to the longer, larger axons that connect various centers of the nervous system: Jacobson's Class I neurons (Jacobson, 1975). Class II neurons have shorter, smaller diameter axons with less myelin and serve mainly to interconnect neurons within a particular brain region (e.g., the cerebral cortex). The "soft wiring" of the nervous system via the Class II neurons may have innate and performance aspects, whereby certain synapses are genetically predetermined and others will be conditioned by particular sensory and motor experience (also see Anokhin, 1964). The full maturation of the "soft wiring" for the speech motor control system may extend to the close of puberty.

Some theorists argue it is the syllable that is the basic programming unit of the speech motor command structure, others maintain these units are smaller than the syllable, whereas some imagine command structures as large as a phrase or sentence (see review in MacNeilage and Ladefoged, 1976). Regardless of the size of the programming unit the child eventually uses in his or her adult nervous system, the basic units of practice (especially in the second year of life) appear to be words (mainly nouns) of rather motorically simple syllable structure. If locomotion practice in the early part of this period is that of the toddler, the speech motor skill might be characterized as that of the wobbler. By the end of this period, most normal children will have produced and practiced many times almost all of the single consonant and vowel combinations of their mother tongue, including some consonant blends and most diphthongs as well. The movements are slower than adults and the durations of consonant and vowel segments are more variable than the adults. This also seems a reasonable time for the child to be learning some of the *gross coordinations* between the functional components. Because the velopharynx, larynx, and lips-tongue-jaw are now moving in concert, it becomes increasingly difficult to judge the functional motor skill of the individual parts by simply listening to the word productions and making some perceptual-phonetic interpretation of the acoustic output. Acoustic studies of this period will help immeasurably, but aerodynamic and movement data should prove to be even more illuminating. If some components develop skill more quickly than others, it may be that the overall coordination of the movements is timed to the less skilled members of the system.

REFINEMENT PERIOD (2 TO 14 YEARS)

If the first 24 months of vocalization and verbalization are thought of as a speech emergence period, the time span of 2 to 14 years might be termed the speech refinement period in terms of speech motor control. Whereas the adult listener may consider most 7 year olds to be adult-like talkers, even the most general studies of speech acoustics show the voice onset times, formant frequencies, and fundamental frequency control are far from adult-like at this time (see review in Kent, 1976).

Neural Maturation. The middle cerebral peduncle is fully myelinated around 3 to 4 years of age and the postthalamic acoustic pathways at 4 to 5 years. The cerebral commissures complete their myelination at about 7 years whereas the secondary association areas continue until the third decade of life, if not longer (Milner, 1976; Yakovlev and Lecours, 1967).

Motor Control. The child begins to adjust consonant and vowel durations to the number of syllables and stressed elements in a phrase or sentence at around 3 to 4 years of age (Kent, 1976). That is, he or she may be beginning to make durational adjustments of the overall motor command structure at about the time the *spatial-temporal coordination* of the speech motor control system is nearing full maturation. The term *spatial-temporal coordination* refers here to the ability to bring the individual component parts to a particular vocal tract *place* or *shape* at a particular *time* to effect critical acoustic events. For example, in producing the syllable *pa*, several structures have to be spatially coordinated at particular *points in time*. Just a few milliseconds prior to lip release for aspiration of the *p*, the velopharynx has to be sealed and the vocal folds have to be abducting, if not fully abducted. The lips, velopharynx, and larynx have to spatially coordinate at this particular time point in order for the aspirated, voiceless *p* to be acoustically realized. The thesis is that the child's earlier speech motor tasks are to build in these spatial-temporal coordinations of the vocal tract. The spatial-temporal coordination of these fundamental movement routines are made with little regard to the total time it takes to execute them or the overall length of the phrase or sentence being produced. As the child increases this spatial-temporal coordination skill, he or she begins to increase the overall execution speed of the motor programs, when the spatial coordination can still be maintained and the various segment durations become conditioned by the linguistic content of the productions. Partial support for this notion is found in the data and interpretation of Gilbert and Purves (1977) for consonant durations in 5- and 7-year-old children. They posit an early "articulation dominant" system followed by a "timing dominant" system (after Ohala, 1970).

NEURAL ORIGINS OF SPEECH MOVEMENTS

The earlier discussion of speech motor control placed it in a unique category of human movement. The search for a particular neuroanatomy that subserves speech movements has remained essentially at the armchair level. The thesis developed in the present chapter is that the neural controls for speech movements are unique to the human and it is hypothesized that an equally particular microneuroanatomy has evolved to control those movements. A corollary to this hypothesis is that speech movements are *not* differentiations, elaborations, or any other form of refinement of more primitive or vegetative processes such as sucking, biting, chewing, or swallowing. This matter has more than theoretical interest since a number of speech therapists reportedly require their clients to practice vegetative movements as necessary prerequisites for the eventual practice of speech production (see reviews in Crickmay, 1977; Fawcus, 1967; Hixon and Hardy, 1964).

One of the central rationales for using "vegetative therapy" is that these nonspeech movements are ontogenic predecessors of speech movements. According to this notion speech is an "overlaid function" on these earlier movement patterns that are the "building blocks" from which speech movements emerge. Several lines of evidence are developed below to hypothesize that speech and vegetative movements are (1) developed *in parallel*; and (2) subserved at least in part by *different* neuronal structures.

Embryonic Differentiation

Yakovlev (1962) uses the "principle of the three-layered structure" in his discussion of human embryologic development. The body representation in the 2-week embryo is in three layers; from inside out, these are labeled the *endoderm, mesoderm,* and *ectoderm.* The internal organs and viscera will grow from the *endoderm,* the musculoskeletal system from the *mesoderm,* and the skin, sense organs, and nervous system from the *ectoderm.*

> The development of the nervous system recapitulates the three-layered plan of the body in the differentiation of neuron aggregates in the three germinal layers of the wall of hollow neuraxis, the innermost or *matrix,* the intermediate or *mantle* and the outermost or *marginal* layers, and anticipates the development of behavior in three space-referred spheres of motility from within out. The matrix layer, nearest the central hollow of the neuraxis, becomes the substratum of the homeostatic regulation of the physiological processes (changes of states) in the internal environment through a diffuse network of neurons that pervade the body and form the short reflex arcs with the peripheral ends sunk deeply in the tissues and organs of the body. The mantle or nuclear layer becomes the substratum of the postural adjustments of the body and its parts to the body itself (changes of form) in all motility of outward (overt) expression of internal states ("emotions") through the nucleated aggregates of neurons which make up longer reflex arcs with the peripheral ends buried in the body wall. The marginal or *cortical* layer, facing the world of objects and of public events about the body, becomes the substratum of translation of the private experience of living into increasing public motility-experience of effective transaction with the external environment (changes of adaptive relations) mainly through the stratilaminate neuronal aggregates of cerebral cortex making up the central ends of long reflex arcs with the peripheral ends cast out into the external environment.
> (Yakovlev, pp. 4–5, 1962)

From these embryologic hypotheses, it seems reasonable to surmise that the neural and musculoskeletal elements that eventually constitute the speech mechanism had their *body* origins in the ectoderm, mesoderm and endoderm. The vegetative movements are hypothesized to have their musculoskeletal origins in the mesoderm and endoderm. The *neural* controls for speech movements are hypothesized to arise from the mantle (nuclear) and marginal (cortical) layers, whereas the neural mechansims that eventually serve vegetative movements originate primarily in the matrix and mantle layers. In short, although the speech and vegetative movements may share certain embryonic origins (e.g., the mesoderm and endoderm of the body, and the mantle or nuclear layer of the nervous system), they also have separate body and nervous system origins in the embryo.

Myelination

There is a centrifugal growth pattern of the myelin (beginning *in utero* in the brainstem) that progresses headward and footward, mostly along a vertical axis (Milner, 1976; Whitaker, 1976). Life begins with the subcortical substrate for the vegetative survival functions (i.e., breathing, sucking, and swallowing). As myelination proceeds to the head and feet, the beginnings of talking and walking, respectively, appear around the end of the first year of life.

Growth and maturation of the cerebral cortex proceeds in a centrifugal pattern and at different rates in particular areas (Milner, 1976; Yakovlev and Lecours, 1967). The primary areas of the visual, motor, somatosensory, and auditory cortices become myelinated in that approximate order to complete a *vertical* "hard wiring" of the long loop, fast-acting pathways toward the end of the first year. Secondary areas and association areas myelinate in a *horizontal* direction as zones around these primary centers. These later horizontal developments are regarded as critical to the eventual development of speech and language and have no known role in the regulation of vegetative movements.

Dendritic Growth

Dendritic bundles have been recommended as storage sites for motor programs or routines (Scheibel, 1979; Scheibel and Scheibel, 1976). These bundles are clustered about cortical motoneurons as well as lower motoneurons. Scheibel and Scheibel (1976) point out that

> The development of these bundles appears, in some cases, to be temporarily correlated with the appearance of certain types of motor output of a stereotyped or repetitive nature, and a putative relationship has been suggested between the two. . . . The dendrite bundle appears to offer a relatively sheltered, and probably specialized, milieu where fragments or whole sequences of stereotyped or repetitive output programs may be coded along the facing membranes of dendrites sprung from the neurons supplying the muscle masses involved. (pp. 242–243)

It is hypothesized that these functional bundles appear as part of the "soft wiring" established for the explicit motor routines of speech. This "plastic" aspect of neural development for speech becomes less flexible as the particular speech movement pattern becomes ingrained. Such inflexibility to speech motor control appears toward the end of the first decade of life when the learning of a second language becomes more difficult and motor patterns of the mother tongue become rather fixed. The fixing of these speech motor patterns thus occurs at a time of fixing of the microneuroanatomy that subserves them.

There is an obvious chicken and egg problem here in determining if the neuroanatomy development leads the emergence of the speech movements or if the speech motor practice evokes the dendritic and axonal growth. A reasonable third hypothesis is that both genetically determined growth and practice of the speech motor skill influence the final "hard wiring" of the speech motor control system.

The Nature of Speech and Vegetative Movements

As with the embryologic and postnatal neural development, there are certain commonalities and differences in speech and vegetative movement patterns. One common feature of both types of movement is that they are highly stereotyped and automated. This has led some people to categorize both activities as "reflexive" and this raises the issue as to whether reflexes are used in speech movements.* Others might contend that reflexes must be inhibited or suppressed in order for normal speech movements to occur. Again, there is a middle ground thesis to suggest we use some reflexive motor patterns that would be competitive with the speech movements. For example, consider the diagram in Figure 1–6. Stimulation to the afferent (trigeminal) nerve evokes two responses (R1 and R2) from the lip muscle (orbicularis oris). The first response is ipsilateral and occurs around 12 ms post stimulus and runs a short peripheral loop through the lower brainstem. R1 is modulated during speech movements but the central versus peripheral contributions to these modulations have yet to be determined (McClean, 1978; Netsell and Abbs, 1975). The second response (R2) is bilateral and has a latency of around 30 to 40 ms and its pathway is less certain. Some contend it runs as high as the motor cortex whereas others maintain the longer delay reflects multiple synapses at the subcortical level (Ekbom, Jernelius, and Kugelberg, 1952). [†] In persons with certain central nervous system pathologies, R2 does not habituate to repeated stimulation and is accompanied by "reflexive" muscle contractions. Such a contrac-

---

*Reflex is defined here as a highly stereotyped response to an adequate stimulus that may or may not be modulated by repeated stimulation.

[†] The eye has R1 and R2 counterparts with R2 being associated with the eye blink.

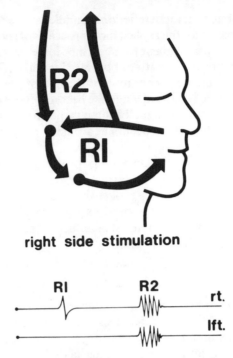

right side stimulation

Figure 1-6. Schematic representation of perioral reflex circuits and the origins of their first and second responses (R1 and R2, respectively).

tion is clearly deleterious to speech movements although some might argue that part or all of the circuitry for R2 is used for speech movements by the neurologically normal talker.

Even though the neural commands for speech and vegetative movements might share certain elements of the schematic circuits shown in Figure 1–6, it is clear that the command centers have different origins *at some place* in the nervous system. From the preceding discussions, it is generally assumed that the speech commands originate in the cerebral cortex and the vegetative commands are triggered from external stimuli or subcortical neurons. Regardless of their loci, the speech and vegetative neural commands are conceived as *parallel* inputs that would *compete* at some level of the neuraxis for the "final" effector neurons if issued *simultaneously*. It follows that the vegetative command neurons might be inhibited or otherwise quieted during speech activity.

Summing Up

Given the embryologic and postnatal neural development reviewed here, the existence of a microneuroanatomy for speech movements seems entirely plausible. Assuming there are motor analogs to the loss of sensory nerve cells due to disuse, the establishment and maintenance of the speech neuroanatomy would seem dependent upon the emergence, refinement, and practice of speech movements. The establishment and practice of vegetative movements as prerequisites or facilitators of speech movements seems counterintuitive to the hypotheses developed in this section. Indeed, the practice of vegetative movements would serve only to facilitate the vegetative synapses that must be inhibited during speech production.

SPEECH MOTOR AGE

It may prove useful to develop a measure of the child's speech motor age (SMA).* Figure 1–7 shows one way to represent such an age, in which the individual functional components (as depicted in Figure 1–1) are assigned a particular month-level based on the child's performance of selected speech motor acts. The acts were selected as a minimal set to represent increasing control of the particular part. Moreover, the speech acts or behaviors shown here are a very preliminary set and were drawn from existing literature, which (for the most part) is based on phonetic transcriptions. A more comprehensive chart is being developed by Morris (1980) that includes developmental aspects of pre-speech activities and feeding as well as vocalizations and verbalizations of the first 24 months.

A more complete speech motor age chart would extend to perhaps 14 years and the long-term goal would be to include speech motor acts that captured the essence of minimal change or development in both the speech emergence and speech refinement periods. It is implicit that the final chart will be built from a large body of perceptual, acoustic, and physiologic data taken from normally developing children. Given these data, it may be possible to assign a fairly well-defined speech motor age to a child. He or she may show a rather uniform delay in motor development across the component parts or differential problems in controlling the parts for speech. Regardless, these speech motor profiles should prove quite useful in implicating or ruling out a neurologic component in to the speech motor output, especially when coupled with electrophysiologic data on the afferent system maturation and the developmental age of other motor systems.

HYPOTHESES ABOUT THE ACQUISTION OF SPEECH MOTOR CONTROL

Throughout this chapter a number of implicit hypotheses have been offered about how the skill of speech motor control might be acquired. It

---

*The author thanks Pamela Boren and Amy Grothman for their assistance in developing this particular chart. It appeared initially in a related representation (Miller, Rosin, and Netsell, 1979).

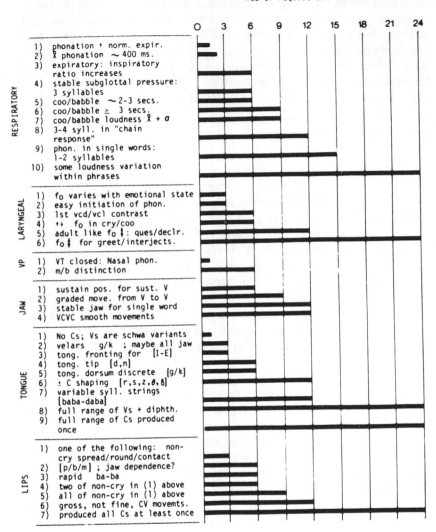

Figure 1-7. A preliminary chart of speech motor milestones in the first two years. Selected speech behaviors are listed for each functional component of the speech mechanism (e.g., 10 behaviors are listed for the respiratory component, six for the laryngeal component, and so forth). From Miller, J., Rosen, R., and Netsell, R. (1979)

may bore the reader and overextend the writer to summarize all those notions at this point, but a few of the more central themes that were developed will be summarized. In each case, the hypothesis and any corollaries are largely unsupported by data, as are hypotheses to the contrary. As a result, I believe they represent important issues around which to build experiments to further our understanding of human language development.

Speech is a motor skill. Speech motor control is an *acquired* motor *skill*. It is *learned* through the *imitation* of *acoustic* patterns provided by an "adult *model*" of the language.

Normal acquisition of speech motor control is dependent on the early establishment of "auditory linkages" and the somatic afferent patterns associated with the emerging speech movements and postures.

Functionally, the neonate is nearly a "subcortical, split-brain organism" in terms of the neural and movement substrate that will serve the acquisition of speech motor control. Accordingly, the vegetative sensorimotor routines used and developed in the neonatal period are *not* the building blocks or "neuromotor foundations" from which speech movements will emerge, differentiate, or otherwise be refined. This hypothesis does not exclude the possibility that speech motor control may not use many of the neonatal nervous system circuits or incorporate elements of certain neonatal "reflexes."

"Sensitive period." A sensitive period for the eventual acquisition of normal speech motor control appears in the postnatal span of 3 to 12 months. This period combines the crucial anatomic developments of the neural and musculoskeletal systems that subserve speech production with the emergence of discrete speech movements along the vocal tract. Failure of the infant to mature at near normal rates in this period will likely place him or her at risk with respect to delays or other abnormalities in speech motor control.

From spatial to temporal control. Speech motor control developed in the first 24 months is dominated by spatial goals in that the child is practicing placement, shaping, or movements of the component parts that yield acoustic patterns to approximate his model(s). *Spatial-temporal coordination*, a "bringing together of selected structures at critical points in time," is dominant in speech motor control over a period of, perhaps, 1 to 6 years. As the child increases this spatial-temporal coordination skill, he or she begins to increase the overall execution speed of the motor programs, in which the spatial coordination can still be maintained and the various segment durations become conditioned by the linguistic content of the productions. This latter time period undoubtedly overlaps the spatial-temporal period, ranging perhaps from 3 to 11 years of chronological age

A continuous process. The acquisition of speech motor skills is a continuous, but nonlinear process. Periods of nonlinearity occur when certain neural, musculoskeletal, environmental, and cognitive changes combine in the individual organism. One such nonlinearity occurs around 1 year of age when marked developments in speech motor control occur with the completion of "hard wiring" of the sensorimotor pathways and a stabilization of musculoskeletal growth.

Optimal behavioral intervention. It is problematic that the child uses "conscious" control of speech movements in learning to talk. He or she may unconsciously develop control of speech movements in a manner similar to the way in which adults unconsciously generate their speech movements. Intervention strategies that bring speech movement routines to a level of visual or kinesthetic awareness may be contrary to these more natural control processes. Optimal behavioral interventions will treat the speech motor control problem at the level it was learned.

From physiology to phonology. The naturalness of fundamental phonetic units (e.g., syllables of CV, VC, and VCV shape) is a "physiologic artifact" of the infant's speech motor capability. The speech motor capability of the first 12 months is influenced most strongly by the status of the child's neurosensorimotor maturation and musculoskeletal system. Similar physiologic influences on phonologic development should be sought for explanations of language development in the second year of life. As stated by Peterson and Shoup (1966), "There is considerable reason to believe that the phonological aspects of speech are primarily organized in terms of the possibilities and constraints of the motor mechanism with which speech is produced" (p. 7).

ACKNOWLEDGMENT

The author wishes to thank Ms. Jan Jensen of the Boys Town National Institute Research staff for editing the manuscript and providing many of the references cited herein. Dr. Josephine Moore (Department of Anatomy, School of Medicine at the University of South Dakota in Vermillion) provided valuable comments on an earlier draft, but is in no way responsible for any inaccuracies of this final form.

REFERENCES

Abbs, J., Muller, E., Hassul, M., and Netsell, R. (1977). *A systems analysis of possible afferent contributions to lip movement control.* Paper presented to American Speech and Hearing Association, Chicago.

Anokhin, P. (1964). Systemogenesis as a general regulator of brain development. In W. Himwich and H. Himwich (Eds.), *The developing brain.* New York: Elsevier, pp. 54–86.

Bosma, J., Truby, H., and Lind, J. (1965). Cry motions of the newborn infant. In J. Lind (Ed.), *Newborn infant cry.* Uppsala: Almqvist and Wiksell.

Bouhuys, A. (1971). Respiration: growth and development. In *Patterns of orofacial growth and development,* ASHA Reports, No. 6, 96–105.

Capute, A., Accardo, P., Vining, E., Rubenstein, J., and Harryman, S. (1978). *Primitive reflex profile: Monographs in developmental pediatrics,* Vol. 1. Baltimore: University Park Press.

Crickmay, M. (1977). *Speech therapy and the Bobath approach to cerebral palsy.* Springfield, IL: Charles C. Thomas.

Desmedt, J. (1978). *Cerebral motor control in man: Long loop mechanism.* Basel: S. Karger.

Ekbom, K., Jernelius, M., and Kugelberg, E. (1952). Perioral reflexes. *Neurology,* 2, 103–111.

Fawcus, R. (1967). Oropharyngeal function in relation to speech. *Developmental Medicine and Child Neurology, 11,* 556–560.

Ferguson, C., and Garnica, O. (1975). Theories of phonological development. In E. Lenneberg and E. Lenneberg (Eds.), *Foundations of language development: A multidisciplinary approach,* Vol. 1. New York: Academic Press, pp. 153–180.

Ferry, P., Culbertson, J., Fitzgibbons, P., and Netzky, M. (1979). Brain function and language disabilities. *Journal of Pediatric Otorhinolaryngology, 1,* 13–24.

Fletcher, S. (1971). Deglutition. In *Patterns of orofacial growth and development,* ASHA Reports, No. 6, 66–78.

Gazzaniga, M. (1970). *The bisected brain.* New York: Appleton.

Gilbert, J., and Purves, B. (1977). Temporal constraints on consonant clusters in child production. *Journal of Child Language, 4,* 417–432.

Hardy, J. (1970). Development of neuromuscular systems underlying speech production. In *Speech and the dentofacial complex: The state of the art.* Asha Reports, No. 5, 49–68.

Hecox, K. (1975). Electrophysiological correlates of human auditory development. In *Infant perception: From sensation to cognition.* Vol. 2, Perception of Space, Speech, and Sound. New York: Academic Press, pp. 151–191.

Hixon, T., and Hardy, J. (1964). Restricted motility of the speech articulators in cerebral palsy. *Journal of Speech and Hearing Disorders, 29,* 293–306.

Humphrey, T. (1971). Human prenatal activity sequences in the facial region and their relationship to postnatal development. In *Patterns of orofacial growth and development,* No. 6, 19–37.

Jacobson, M. (1975). Brain development in relation to language. In E. Lenneberg and E. Lenneberg (Eds.), *Foundations of language development: A multidisciplinary approach,* Vol. 1. New York: Academic Press, pp. 105–120.

Kent, R. (1976). Anatomical and neuromuscular maturation of the speech mechanism: Evidence from acoustic studies. *Journal of Speech and Hearing Research, 19,* 422–447.

Kent, R.D. (1981). Articulatory acoustic perspectives on speech development. In R. Stark (Ed.), *Language behavior in infancy and early childhood.* New York: Elsevier/North Holland, pp. 105–126.

Kent, R., and Minifie, F. (1977). Coarticulation in recent speech production models. *Journal of Phonetics, 5*(2), 115–133.

Kent, R., and Moll, K. (1975). Articulatory timing in selected consonant sequences. *Brain Language, 2,* 304–323.

Ladefoged, P., DeClerk, J., Lindau, M., and Papcun, G. (1972). An auditory-motor theory of speech production. UCLA Working Papers in Phonetics, No. 22, 48–75.

Langlois, A., and Baken, R. (1976). Development of respiratory time-factors in infant cry. *Developmental Medicine and Child Neurology, 18,* 732–737.

Lecours, A. (1975). Myelogenetic correlates of the development of speech and language. In E. Lenneberg and E. Lenneberg (Eds.), *Foundations of language development: A multidisciplinary approach,* Vol. 1, New York: Academic Press, pp. 121–136.

Lindblom, B., Lubker, J., and Gay, T. (1979). Formant frequencies of some fixed-mandible vowels and a model of speech motor programming by predictive simulation. *Journal of Phonetics, 7,* 147–161.

McClean, M. (1978). Variation in perioral reflex amplitude prior to lip muscle contraction for speech. *Journal of Speech and Hearing Research, 21,* 276–284.

MacNeilage, P., and Ladefoged, P. (1976). The production of speech and language. In E. Carterette and M. Friedman (Eds.), *Handbook of perception,* Volume VII, Language and Speech, New York: Academic Press, pp. 75–120.

Miller, J., Rosin, P., and Netsell, R. (1979). *Differentiating productive language deficits and speech motor control problems in children.* Paper presented at the meeting of the Wisconsin Speech and Hearing Association, Madison, WI

Milner, E. (1976). CNS maturation and language acquisition. In H. Whitaker and H. A. Whitaker (Eds.), *Studies in neurolinguistics,* Vol. 1. New York: Academic Press, pp. 31–102.

Morris, S. (1980). Pre-speech assessment scale: A rating scale for the measurement of the pre-speech behaviors from birth through two years. *Experimental Edition,* Curative Rehabilitation Center, Milwaukee, WI.

Moyers, R. (1971). Postnatal development of the orofacial musculature. In *Patterns of orofacial growth and development,* ASHA Reports, No. 6, 38–47.

Nakazima, S. (1975). Phonemicization and symbolization in language development. In E. Lenneberg and E. Lenneberg (Eds.), *Foundations of language development: A multidisciplinary approach,* Vol. 1. New York: Academic Press, pp. 181–188.

Netsell, R., and Abbs, J. (1975). Modulation of perioral reflex sensitivity during speech movements. *Journal of the Acoustical Society of America,* Supp. S41.

Netsell, R., Kent, R., and Abbs, J. (1978). *Adjustments of the tongue and lips to fixed jaw positions during speech: A preliminary report.* Paper presented to the Conference on Speech Motor Control, University of Wisconsin, Madison.

Ohala, J. (1970). Aspects of the control and production of speech. *UCLA Working Papers on Phonetics,* No. 15.

Oller, K. (1978). The emergence of the sounds of speech in infancy. In the Proceedings of the NICHD Conference on *Child Phonology: Perception, Production, and Deviation,* Bethesda, MD, May 28-31.

Peterson, G., and Shoup, J. (1966). A physiologic theory of phonetics. *Journal of Speech and Hearing Research, 9,* 5–67.

Porter, R. (1978). *Rapid shadowing of syllables: Evidence for symmetry of speech perceptual and motor systems.* Presented at the 19th Annual Meeting of the

Psychonomic Society, San Antonio, Texas, November 9-11.

Porter, R.J., and Castellanos, F.X. (1980). Speech production-measures of speech perception: Rapid shadowing of VCV syllables. *Journal of the Acoustical Society of America, 67,* 1349–1356.

Porter, R.J., and Lubker, J.F. (1980). Rapid reproduction of vowel-vowel sequences: Evidence for a fast direct acoustic-motoric linkage. *Journal of Speech and Hearing Research, 23,* 593–603.

Rutherford, D. (1967). Auditory-motor learning and the acquisition of speech. *American Journal of Physical Medicine, 46,* 245–251.

Scheibel, A. (1979). Development of axonal and dendritic neuropil as a function of evolving behavior. In F.O. Schmitt and F.G. Worden (Eds.), *The neurosciences fourth study program.* Cambridge, MA: MIT Press, pp. 381–398.

Scheibel, M., and Scheibel, A. (1976). Some thoughts on the ontogeny of memory and learning. In M. Rosenzweig and E. Bennet (Eds.), *Neural mechanisms of learning and memory.* Cambridge, MA: MIT Press.

Shirley, M. (1959). *The first two years.* Volume 1: Postural and Locomotor Developments. Minneapolis: University of Minnesota Press.

Sloan, R. (1967). Neuronal histogenesis, maturation and organization related to speech development. *Journal of Communication Disorders, 1,* 1–15.

Stark, R., and Nathanson, S. (1973). Spontaneous cry in the newborn infant: Sounds and facial gestures. In J. Bosma (Ed.), *Fourth symposium on oral sensation and perception: Development in the fetus and infant.* Washington, DC: Report DHEW (NIH) 73–546, Superintendent of Documents.

Weiffenbach, J., and Thach, B. (1973). Elicited tongue movements: Touch and tests in the newborn human. In J. Bosma (Ed.), *Fourth symposium on oral sensation and perception: Development in the fetus and infant.* Washington, DC: Report DHEW (NIH) 73-546, Superintendent of Documents.

Whitaker, H. (1976). Neurobiology of language. In E. Carterette and M. Friedman (Eds.), *Handbook of perception,* Volume VII, Language and speech. New York: Academic Press, pp. 121–144.

Wilder, C., and Baken, R. (1974, Winter). Respiratory patterns in infant cry. *Human Communication,* pp. 18–34.

Wilder, C., and Baken, R. (1978). Some developmental aspects of infant cry. *Journal of Genetic Psychology, 132,* 225–230.

Wolff, P. (1969). The natural history of crying and other vocalizations in early infancy. In F. Foss (Ed.), *Determinants of infant behavior,* Volume IV. London: Methuen & Co.

Woodruff, D. (1978). Brain electrical activity and behavior relationships over the life span. In P. Bates (Ed.), *Life span development and behavior,* Vol. I. New York: Academic Press.

Yakovlev, P. (1962). Morphological criteria of growth and maturation of the nervous system in man. In L. Kolb, R. Masland, and R. Cooke (Eds.), *Mental retardation.* Research in Nervous and Mental Disease, Vol. XXXIX.

Yakovlev, P., and Lecours, A. (1967). The myelogenetic cycles of regional maturation of the brain. In A. Minkowski (Ed.), *Regional development of the brain in early life.* Oxford, England: Blackwell Scientific Publications.

Chapter *2*

Speech Motor Control and Selected Neurologic Disorders

The primary purpose of this chapter is to recruit basic and clinical neuroscientists to the study of speech motor control and its disorders. The topics below are briefly reviewed to acquaint these potential colleagues with one person's view of (1) speech as a motor control system and (2) selected problems of "dyscontrol" that result from nervous system damage.

It is emphasized that the ideas presented range from notions to hypotheses and, as such, represent only beginning points for discussion and the design of experiments.

SPEECH AS A MOTOR CONTROL SYSTEM

Language is said to have evolved as a communication system to interface "man's intellect with his peripheral apparatus" (Studdert-Kennedy, 1980). Speech is the motor-acoustic expression of language and speech

Reprinted by permission of the publisher from *Speech motor control*, S. Grillner, B. Lindblom, J. Lubker, and A. Persson (Eds.). Proceedings of an International Symposium on the Functional Basis of Oculomotor Disorders, pp. 247–261. Copyright 1982 by Pergamon Press, Inc., New York.

33

motor control is defined here as the motor-afferent mechanisms that direct and regulate speech movements. *Mechanisms* refer to the muscle and neural anatomy and physiology that have evolved for the purpose of producing speech movements (i.e., the purposive movements for generating the unique acoustic patterns of a particular language). The afferent mechanisms believed essential to normal speech motor control are auditory and somatoafferent (Fig. 2–1). Somato*afferent*, as used here, includes all information arising from the musculoskeletal system during posture and movement.

Given the foregoing definitions, the matter of *formulating* a given spoken message is excluded from the domain of speech motor control. The concepts of cognition and language (involved in ideation, intention, comprehension, planning, and the like) and their neuronal representations are not considered in detail here. Communication disorders of these meta-speech processes are the problems of aphasia (dysphasia) and apraxia (dyspraxia). Speech disorders of motor control, as defined earlier, are referred to collectively as the *dysarthrias* (see Darley, Aronson, and Brown, 1975). These dysphasia, dyspraxia, and dysarthria distinctions have clinical reality in that they often appear as separate entities. However, more often than not, these neurogenic communication disorders coexist, and selective damage to their respective neurologic representations is probably very rare, considering the evolution of the human nervous system presented later in this chapter.

Evolutionary Influences

In looking to nonhuman primates for clues about the origins of human speech motor control, the evolution of the entire nervous system is considered as well as the more recent neocortical development.

Ethologic Considerations. It is suggested that the human brain evolved from more primitive forms, with residuals of the reticular and limbic nervous systems having served as whole brains for reptiles and monkeys, respectively (see reviews in Ploog, 1979; Robinson, 1976; Steklis and Raleigh, 1979). Even though monkeys developed a neocortical system, their vocalizations (however purposive in intent) are believed to use the limbic system only (Ploog, 1979; Sutton, Larson, and Lindeman, 1974). Although we accept that monkeys and apes do think, have language, and express both in their vocalizations, their quantity (if not quality) is far inferior to human. It is doubtful that the nonhuman primates' limitations with speech motor control are musculoskeletal or neuronal per se. More likely their limitations are cognitive and the human-nonhuman differences in complexity of communication skill are solely attributable to neocortical

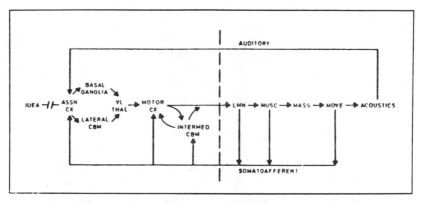

Figure 2-1. Diagrammatic representation of neural pathways, modules, and the musculoskeletal system hypothesized to be used in the motor control of speech (composite drawing adapted from Allen and Tsukahara, 1974; Grimm and Nashner, 1978). Vertical dashed line separates peripheral (right side) and central (left side) nervous systems. CX, Cortex; CBM, Cerebellum; LMN, lower motoneurons; MUSC, muscles; MOVE, movements.

system developments, including the hemispheric dominance of the human (Ploog, 1979; Steklis and Raleigh, 1979; Studdert-Kennedy, 1980).

Neocortical system development is not restricted to cerebral cortex elaboration. Additional allometric changes in cerebellum, corpus striatum, and thalamus are regarded as central to the human neocortical system and the associated motor skills. Even though the neocortical system dominates more primitive centers, the phylogenetically older limbic communication systems remain and often dominate following certain neurologic lesions (Kornhuber, 1977; Ploog, 1979; Robinson, 1976). It is emphasized that both human language and speech are strongly represented at subcortical as well as cortical levels and that the homologues of the older reticular and limbic systems eventually may be shown to exert more than general arousal and emotional effects on human communication.

It is speculated that the neocortical system has evolved to meet the increased needs and demands for control through action (i.e., as the most overt expression of human intelligence) (Granit, 1977; Kornhuber, 1977). Such fine motor skill is most elaborately demonstrated in playing the violin or piano, or in the physical act of speaking. Some of the pathways believed involved in these skills are shown in the central nervous system representations of Figure 2–1. In this scheme, the motor cortex is a summing point that has been likened to a "somatic association area, a specialized tool of tactile and proprioceptive adjustments for those movements that specifically require this kind of regulation" (Kornhuber, 1977). The hypothesized contributions of these neocortical regions and pathways in normal human motor control, including speech, have been reviewed elsewhere (Abbs and

Cole, 1982; Desmedt, 1978; Evarts, 1982; Persson, 1979).

In terms of formulating and initiating speech and language, Broca's and Wernicke's areas presumably are the critical association cortices (ASSN CX in Fig. 2–1). Again, subcortical influences are strong, with limbic-to-frontal-to-Broca connections in the precentral regions and limbic-to-temporal and parietal-to-Wernicke in the postcentral regions (Kornhuber, 1977). Recent electrical stimulation experiments suggest Broca's area as a "final motor pathway for speech," with strong and reciprocal connections to parietal areas involved in "sequencing movement and phonemic discrimination" (Ojemann and Mateer, 1980). As suggested in Figure 2–1, *both* Broca's and Wernicke's areas have inputs to the basal ganglia and, via pontine nuclei, the cerebellum.

Speech as a Motor Skill

In speech, as with other motor control skills, the most fundamental questions are "What is being *controlled* (directed)?" and "What is doing the *controlling* (regulating)?" Concerning the latter, combinations of "elementary units of behavior" (e.g., reflexes, servomechanisms, and oscillators) have been used to describe apparently complex behaviors in lower animals (see review in Gallistel, 1980; Grillner, 1982). It is conceivable that the discovery of a few additional units ("a number nearer 10 than 100," Gallistel, 1980) will be useful in conceptualizing the *regulatory* mechanisms of speech motor control.

A central related issue concerns the extent to which different "*units of behavior*" are recruited for the various speech and vegetative motor tasks of the same musculoskeletal structures. For example, the gag and swallow reflexes are inhibited or suppressed during speech production and it is doubtful that elements of them are somehow selectively recruited for speech purposes. It is hypothesized that specialized neuronal "connectivities" (after Scheibel, 1979) and patterns of muscle activation are developed for the motor skill of speech (see Chapter 1 and Hixon and Hardy, 1964). A corollary of this hypothesis is that *speech movements* must be practiced so that these neuronal and muscle activations be realized. There presently exists no experimental evidence that vegetative patterns are prerequisites for speech motor control or that their practice will facilitate the emergence of speech movements, even though some clinicians advocate this type of practice.

Concerning "*what* is being controlled (directed)," it also is likely that the mode, or strategy (i.e., pattern), of control to the same musculoskeletal structures varies with the movement requirements (i.e., the goals attempted)

(Granit, 1977; Gurfinkel and Levik, 1979).

Speech production meets the general requirements of a fine motor skill: (1) it is performed with accuracy and speed, (2) it uses knowledge of results, (3) it is improved by practice, (4) it demonstrates motor flexibility in achieving goals, and (5) it relegates all of this to automatic control, where "consciousness" is freed from the details of action plans (Wolff, 1979). As a motor skill, speech is goal-directed and afferent-guided. The goal is to produce the appropriate acoustic patterns via flexible motor *actions* that are formed and maintained by "auditory images." These auditory images, in turn, become yoked to the motor and somatoafferent patterns used to generate them (see Wolff's discussion of perceptual motor ideas). These ideas are highly similar to those of others (cf. Bernshtein, 1967; Gurfinkel and Levik, 1979; Hardy, 1971; Ladefoged, DeClerk, Lindau, and Papcun, 1972; MacNeilage, 1970).

It is underscored that these motor *actions* are not fixed movement routines or stored patterns of muscle contractions. The speaker can employ a highly flexible motor program to achieve a highly consistent acoustic product. His or her internal referent is what it feels and sounds like to produce certain speech movements and acoustics. Similarly, the "proficient violinist breaks a string while playing a recital but continues the performance without interruption by reprogramming the usual fingering, and playing the required notes on different strings. The 'motor idea' controlling the musical performance does not prescribe a fixed relation between notes and finger movements, but enables the performer to generate functionally equivalent new finger sequences that will all preserve the musical passage" (Wolff, 1979). Comparable skills are evidenced in speech production (see review in Abbs and Cole, 1982).

Adult-like use of speech acoustics and motor control is not achieved until around the end of the first decade of life (Kent, 1976). It is hypothesized that neural and musculoskeletal developments are continuous through this period, with early emphasis on achieving the spatial aspects of the motor-acoustic goals, and later emphasis on optimizing the speaking rate (Netsell, 1981). It is not clear when children have developed (1) speech "motor ideas," with the full flexibility of motor skill to carry out the demands for action, or (2) the cerebral dominance that controls these neuromotor mechanisms. Preliminary data suggest that the precision of lip motor control in speech is markedly increased between the ages of seven and ten (Watkin and Fromm, in press), and that 10-year-old children do not yet have adult-like gEMG activity of the velum during speech (Lubker, Kuehn, and Fritzell, 1981). It also has been hypothesized that normal children already have cerebral dominance of speech output by age of 3 (White and Kinesbourne, 1980).

Normal Speech Motor Control

In contrast to limb movements, speech movements are made almost entirely within the head, neck, and torso, an exception being the lips' occasional protrusion into the environment of perhaps 5 mm or so. Movements of a single part (e.g., the velum or jaw) are seldom beyond 1 cm, and jaw movements of about 1.5 cm represent an extreme. Typical velocities are in the 5 to 20 cm/s range, with up to 30 cm/s seen in fast movements. When expressed as degrees/second, normal jaw movements during speech are only 15 degrees/s, with maximum speeds around 30 degrees/s. In contrast, fast eye movements and associated head turning are 300 and 200 degrees/s, respectively (Lennerstrand and Bach-y-Rita, 1975).

Whole muscle contractions (as estimated from gross EMG, or gEMG, patterns) typically are 75 to 100 ms duration for simple, unidirectional movements (as in elevating the lower lip to make a *p* sound). Given the foregoing values, conversational rates of speech occur at about 4 syllables/s, as in counting aloud "one thousand one, one thousand two," and so on. Unlike the limb muscles acting on a joint, gEMG activity seen during speech movements often lacks clear reciprocal patterning. For example, orbicularis oris may show reciprocal actions with depressor labii inferior in closing and opening movements of the lips for *p* or *b* but show nonreciprocal activity in rounding the lips for *u* or *w*.

The temporal precision in coordinating two parts (e.g., tongue release for *s* and lip closure for *p*) can be as fine as 10 sm (Kent and Moll, 1975). Spatial precision in repeated positioning of the tongue to produce the *ee* sound is within 1 mm (Gay, Lindblom, and Lubker, 1981; Netsell, Kent, and Abbs, 1980).

Muscle contractile forces during speech movements have not been measured directly. Such measurements obviously are necessary to further specify the nature of speech movements. Estimates from indirect sources place muscle forces for speech between 5 and 20 percent of the muscle's maximum isometric force. The force may develop fully within 50 ms, yielding rates of force development in the range of perhaps 0.5 to 2.0 kg/s. This would place speech movements at the low to middle area of the "force ramp" range and not in the "ballistic" category (Desmedt and Godaux, 1978). It is emphasized that these are gross estimates and direct measurements are needed.

Published anatomic studies of motor unit or muscle fiber types in muscles used for speech are few (see exception in Vignon, Pellissier, and Serratrice, 1980). However, given the velocity and force estimates noted earlier, it is predicted that fast contracting, fatigue resistant motor units (type FR in Burke, 1980) predominate for speech purposes. The smallest diameter muscle fibers (type II in Vignon et al., 1980) are postulated as the primary type used in chewing. To meet the various motor task demands on these muscles (e.g., sucking, chewing, swallowing, speaking), highly specialized muscle fiber and neural substrates may have evolved (see Chapter 1 and Dubner, Sessle, and Storey, 1978). That is, "any speculation on neural control mechanisms needs to begin with consideration of the *properties of the motor organ* to be controlled as well as the *nature of the task* being controlled." It is further suggested that "where structural substrates and functional demands vary across different motor organs one might profitably look for *unique neural control organizations*," and "delineation of the ways in which *speech* as a motor task *differs from nonspeech* activities of the same musculature is crucial to the development of valid theories of speech motor control" (italics added) (Bowman, personal communication).

From the foregoing speculations concerning structure and function, it is hypothesized that speech motor control falls between the extremes of extraocular (Lennerstrand and Bach-y-Rita, 1975) and forearm motor control, resembling most closely the fine motor control of the hands and fingers in playing the violin or piano. The full range of movements is made with slow to moderate velocities under highly precise spatial and temporal control. Slow to intermediate force ramps, developed by small to intermediate sized motoneurons and muscle fibers, are good candidates as the muscle force generators. It is further speculated that these characteristics have evolved to allow the system continuous access to its rich somatoafferent feedback, in which the overall speaking rate pushes the upper limit of musculoskeletal response.

SELECTED DISORDERS OF SPEECH MOTOR CONTROL

When particular neural pathways, modules, or regions are damaged, the motor control of speech becomes disrupted. Some of these disruptions are so severe as to render the speech unintelligible. The trained listener can perceptually identify certain speech and voice characteristics as belonging to a person with a given neurologic disorder (see Darley et al., 1975). Only in the past 10 years or so have studies begun to focus on the deviant acoustic, movement, and gEMG patterns associated with the various forms of dysarthria. The selective review that follows will cast these more recent acoustic-physiologic studies against gEMG and single motor unit (SMU) data from limb motor control studies of humans with similar neurologic signs or disease.

Disorders of Muscle Forcing Functions

At the more peripheral levels the motor control problems of the dysarthrias can be viewed as disorders of muscle forcing functions. A *muscle forcing function* is defined here as the *force ramp* (change in force/ change in time, or rate of force, after Desmedt and Godaux, 1978). For simplicity, muscle forcing functions will be discussed in terms of the (1) combined force of prime mover and its agonists, and, when it applies, (2) collective force generated by antagonists. At any one time, the desired, net contractile force of the muscles aiding or opposing the movement is not achieved. Underlying these abnormal muscle forcing functions, of course, is a pathologic recruitment or firing rate of motor units. This concept applies not only to simple movements, such as elevating the velum, but also to (1) the coordination of all muscle forces involved in changing the vocal tract shape during speech and (2) maintaining the overall posture and background stiffness (tonicity) in the muscles.

With respect to generating phasic muscle contractions, the problems are in *specifying* (i.e., turning on, grading, or turning off) and *organizing* these muscle forces, not in selecting the proper muscles (after Weiss in Granit, 1977). For the dysarthrias, in general, the attempts at phasic contractions are weak and slow in developing, and the velocity of movements is reduced. In an exception to be discussed later, speech movements of some dysarthric subjects with Parkinson's disease are made faster than normal.

The problems with phasic muscle forces can be compounded by background tonic contractions in prime movers, agonists, or antagonists that are excessive (hypertonic), reduced (hypotonic), or variable (fluctuating). This excessive or fluctuating stiffness can slow or, in extreme cases, stop a movement.

Tremors are most obvious in vocal folds, where their frequency is audible in the voice. Other rhythmic muscle contractions are not perceived as such but can severely disrupt the generation of muscle force.

Problems and Purposes in Classification

To a large extent, the way in which dysarthrias are classified depends on the purpose of classification. Until recently, neurologists and other clinical researchers have used largely *nosologic* criteria, such as neurologic signs, diseases, and locus of lesion. The nosologic model has guided earlier speech research as well, with the dysarthrias associated with ataxia, Parkinson's disease, and cerebral palsy reflecting the mixed designations of neurologic sign and disease. *Physiologic* criteria recently have been used in the description and habilitation of individual dysarthrics, and combined forms of nosologic-physiologic classifications prevail in most basic and applied studies of these speech disorders. Some advantages of physiologic classification for understanding and treating the dysarthrias will be discussed in a later section.

Representative Forms of Dysarthria

The dysarthrias reviewed in this chapter were chosen for one or more of the following reasons: (1) they are perceptually, acoustically, and physiologically quite distinct from one another; (2) their nervous system loci are reasonably well established; (3) the presumed lesions involve most of the regions or pathways believed to be used in speech motor control; and (4) data on limb motor control problems associated with these lesions are available for comparison.

Dysarthria and Peripheral Lesions. Lesions affecting the peripheral nervous system (see Fig. 2–1), especially the cranial nuclei or nerves, yield a dysarthria that appears relatively straightforward in terms of the speech pattern and presumed motor control problem. The speech is perceived as slow, hypernasal, and breathy, with reduced loudness and reduced pitch variability. These dimensions vary rather predictably with the nuclei and nerves involved. Darley and others (1975) refer to them collectively as "flaccid dysarthrias."

The resulting movements are uniformly slow, but the full range of movement is reached if sufficient muscle force is preserved and applied to the individual movements. If a given component is more severely involved than others (e.g., the velopharynx), the speaker may slow other movements to maintain the coordination and speech intelligibility.

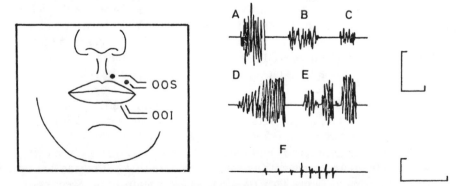

Figure 2–2. Muscle action potentials from orbicularis oris superior (OOS) or inferior (OOI) to close the lips for the sounds *p* and *b*. A, normal; B, reduced amplitude; C, reduced amplitude and duration; D, megaphonic; E, bursting; F, accelerating. Calibration: A–F, 400 microvolts and 100 ms.

The gEMG patterns typically are reduced in amplitude and somewhat shorter than normal duration (compare patterns A, B, and C in Fig. 2–2). No SMU data recorded during speech have been reported for the peripheral dysarthria or for any other form of dysarthria for that matter. From SMU recordings of first dorsal interosseous muscle (Milner-Brown, Stein, and Lee, 1974a, 1974b), normal patterns of recruitment are seen with LMN disease, nerve pressure, or nerve entrapment, but their twitch tension is reduced even when gEMG amplitudes are normal or increased. In severed nerves that have regenerated, normal isometric force is regained even though normal recruitment patterns are not, and problems with fine motor control may persist. Some of the reduced SMU control and force capability may be related to reduced afferent information, because the range of SMU firing rate is affected by afferent nerve deprivation (Grimby and Hannerz, 1979). Reductions in CNS and peripheral facilitation of the lower motoneurons can produce a hypotonicity. These slack muscles also can retard the generation of rapid force increases for speech. The net effect of these peripheral lesions on the muscle forcing function of the prime movers may be to act as a pathologic "low pass filter," whereby motor units of higher firing frequency and amplitude are limited in their influence on the fiber twitches (see also Scott, 1975).

Assuming an intact CNS, most of the normal motor flexibility is available to reorganize the muscle actions to meet the acoustic demands. The extent to which the central adaptive mechanisms can be effective depends on which cranial nerves or nuclei are involved and the severity of their impairment.

Dysarthria and Cerebellar Disorders. Lesions affecting the cerebellum or its connections via the cerebellar peduncles yield a very distinct dysarthria called "ataxic dysarthria" (see reviews in Darley et al., 1975; Kent, Netsell, and Abbs, 1979). The speakers sound inebriated, with all syllables being of similar duration and the pitch of the voice being more variable than normal. Special difficulty arises in articulating sounds that require nearly continuous movement for their perception, such as *r, l,* and diphthongs (e.g., the *oi* in *boil*).

In terms of speech movements, the most striking deficit is the reduction in velocity (Kent and Netsell, 1975; Netsell and Kent, 1976). Even though the movements are slow, and rather uniformly slow, the subjects with cerebellar disorders cannot voluntarily speed up and may be moving as fast as they can. In general, their movements are 1½ to 2 times as slow as those of normal persons. They preserve the gross features of speech coordination but exhibit small timing errors (e.g., between lip, larynx, and velopharynx movements) that distort sound productions. Lesser problems are seen in the range and direction of movement, which are more variable than those of normal subjects in repeating the same words or sentences. The perceptions of subjects with cerebeller disorders of their speech motor problems can be very telling. One woman complained that she "couldn't always make them [the tongue, lips, etc.] go where she wanted them to go," and another ataxic person said he now had to think very carefully about everything he was trying to say.

Two gEMG patterns characterize the available data recorded during speech from cerebellar subjects (Abbs, Barlow, and Cole, 1979; Netsell and Abbs, 1977). One pattern shows a gradual build-up of activity, reaching normal amplitudes toward the latter half to one third of its duration. Once peaked, the gEMG does not quickly reduce, thus prolonging the muscle contraction (Fig. 2–2, D). As with the movements, the gEMG patterns typically are 1½ to 2 times the duration of normal patterns for closing the lips in *p* and *b* sound productions. The second pattern (Fig. 2–2, E) shows multiple bursts of excitation and quieting. These repetitive bursts have a period of approximately 50 to 75 ms and are similar to those seen in the biceps of cerebellar subjects during forearm flexion (Abbs et al., 1979; Terzuolo and Viviani, 1974). These bursts generate fluctuations in force between the lips as the subject tries to make lip closures. In short, the cerebellar subject is slow, or slow plus irregular, in building up the requisite muscle force in the prime mover and, once the force is achieved, cannot rapidly suppress the activity. It also has been hypothesized that cerebellar hypotonia adds to the problems of generating phasic muscle force increases (Gilman, 1969, 1974; Glaser, 1963; Kent and Netsell, 1975).

The motor unit problems underlying these muscle force deficits have not been reported for phasic contractions. In trying to sustain SMU firings at low force levels, ataxic subjects occasionally recruited phasic units, especially following involuntary loss of control in the unit already recruited (Grimby and Hannerz, 1975).

The motor control problems secondary to cerebellar lesions are not well explained by current interpretations. The data are sparse and have been drawn from a variety of subjects with ataxic signs and multiple, suspected, or undefined causes (including brainstem or cerebellar tumor, alcoholism, multiple sclerosis, idiopathic). The dysarthria studies to date reveal more about what the cerebellum *does not* do during speech than what its normal functions might be. If there are no truly ballistic speech movements, the cerebellum is not a pulse or step function generator (Kornhuber, 1974). Moreover, its role seems not central to muscle *selection*, and it would appear to be properly placed peripheral to the demands of association cortices (see Fig. 2–1). A fundamental cerebellar deficit is in grading the development of muscle force, perhaps in response to the demands of the *entire system*. Assuming it is normally somewhat assisting in the time-continuous muscle force specifications, cerebellar failure slows, or makes discontinuous, the normally phasic and precise muscle forces. As a consequence, all muscle contractions tend to have a uniformly long duration, yielding slow velocities to all movements and uniform duration to the syllables. The ability to make shortened, or unstressed, syllables is lost.

It is further speculated that the intermediate zone of cerebellum (see Fig. 2–1) performs a continuous computation on motor cortex output and peripheral inputs so that "movement is being updated *as it is evolving* through a modification of command signals before they impinge on lower motoneurons" (Bowman, personal communication). This capability suggests the cerebellum has the additional role of *velocity adjustor* by making rapid adjustments in the muscle forcing functions. In short, normal cerebellar function keeps individual and collective muscle contractions on schedule, revising motoneuron outputs according to the (1) output goals, and (2) status of the periphery, as signaled by the somatoafference.

Dysarthria with Parkinson's Disease. Persons with Parkinson's disease present a variety of movement disorders throughout the various motor systems. There is a great apparent heterogeneity in both the limb motor problems and speech abnormalities associated with this disease. Most common to all dysarthric persons with parkinsonism is a reduced loudness and a unique voice quality that has yet to be well described in perceptual or acoustic dimensions (Darley et al., 1975; Kent and Netsell, 1979). Some persons with parkinsonian dysarthria speak slowly, some very rapidly, and others have special difficulty in initiating speech. Another remarkable aspect is the great fluctuation in intelligibility. At one moment the speech may be totally unintelligible and in the next it is essentially normal. These problems have not been shown to vary as a function of stage or duration of the disease or age of the speaker (Netsell, 1979; Quaglieri and Celesia, 1977). One study, however, reports that the speech patterns may reflect progressive involvement, beginning in the larynx and extending upward through the upper airway (Logemann, Fisher, Boshes, and Blonsky, 1978).

Clinical observations suggest parkinsonian individuals may have (1) normal or reduced range of movement, (2) decreased, increased, or normal velocity of movement, and (3) direction and coordination of movement within normal limits. Preliminary data with three parkinsonian subjects show a direct relationship between rigidity (resistance to passive movement) and reductions in the range and velocity of lip movements during speech (Hunker, Abbs, and Barlow, 1980). Furthermore, it is suggested that rigidity can be uneven in the facial muscles, as one subject showed considerable increased stiffness in the lower lip and near normal levels in the upper lip. Although cause-effect relations between rigidity and hypokinesia have yet to be established, it was noted that the range and velocity of lower lip movement in this subject were more reduced than they were in the upper lip. In the only other study to quantify speech movements in this disease, the lower lips of two parkinsonian subjects were shown to reach peak accelerations of 200 to 800 cm/s^2, or ten- to 40-fold greater than normal (Marquardt, 1973).

Evidence for both rigidity and acceleration has been demonstrated in gEMG patterns from the facial muscles. Heightened activity has been recorded in muscles antagonistic to lip closing movements, as in forming a *p* or *b* sound (Hunker et al., 1980; Leanderson, Meyerson, and Persson, 1971, 1972). An overall reduction in this excessive gEMG activity was noted following L-dopa administration (Leanderson et al., 1972). These observations fit the hypothesis that reduced range and velocity of movement are related to heightened gEMG in muscles antagonistic to the intended movement. Recordings from orbicularis oris superior muscle in other parkinsonian subjects reveal additional gEMG abnormalities (Netsell, 1979; Netsell, Daniel, and Celesia, 1975). The reduced gEMG amplitude pattern of shortened duration (Fig. 2–2, C) frequently was seen in these subjects, especially those who had undergone thalamic surgery for the relief of rigidity and tremor in the limbs. In other subjects, small amplitude, increasingly rapid gEMG bursts preceded lip closures, with syllable rates reaching as high as 13/s (see Fig. 2–2, F). These rates far exceed normal capabilities and the subjects appear to be in a mode over which they have no immediate control. Interestingly, by increasing loudness or speaking effort, these subjects could override this "acceleration" phenomenon.

Electrophysiologic studies of the extremities offer some clues as to the nature of motor disorders in parkinsonian dysarthria. When attempting to activate SMUs at low force levels, these subjects often have difficulty initiating, sustaining, or shutting down the firing of individual units (Grimby and Hannerz, 1974; Milner-Brown, Fisher, and Weiner, 1979; Petajan and Jarcho, 1975). A problem in motor unit recruitment order has been hypothesized to reflect a "decreased ability to switch from tonic to phasic recruitment order, and vice-versa" (Grimby and Hannerz, 1974). Units recruited with more than minimal muscle contractions often tend to fire in small groups at tremor frequency (Petajan and Jarcho, 1975). This may bear some relation to the acceleration seen with the small gEMG bursts that can be obviated by more effortful muscle contractions. Studies of long latency responses in forearms and thumbs of parkinsonian individuals reveal problems with heightened gEMG in the 50 to 100 ms interval following an abrupt mechanical stimulus (Lee and Tatton, 1978; Mortimer and Webster, 1978). These responses are more exaggerated if a voluntary flexion response is to follow the stimulus. Interestingly, the periods of the 10 to 13 Hz acceleration frequencies seen in speech are approximately 75 to 100 ms. Perhaps in initiating muscle contractions for speech, the small to moderate sized units fire at or near tremor frequency, and these are somehow enhanced, or not inhibited, by the hyperactive long loop responses, leading to the uncontrolled "fast rushes of speech." In this mode the muscles cannot respond fast enough, and the speech becomes an unintelligible blur. In speaking with greater "effort," larger units are recruited more quickly, speech is slowed to syllable rates below the tremor frequency, and the "phase locking" of speech syllable rate to the pathologic tremor is avoided. Rigidity could be exaggerated at slower speech rates, especially during the flexion of orbicularis oris muscle for lip closures, when the more forceful contractions are associated with heightened long loop responses and associated gEMG activity.

Taken together, the foregoing speculations may account for part of the apparent paradoxical existence of akinesia, rigidity, tremor, and "short rushes of speech," or what has been referred to here as "acceleration." The unifying problem may be the "inability to adjust a level of motoneuron facilitation from either one level to another or from an active (zero) state to activity" (Petajan and Jarcho, 1975). In turn, the more central problem may be in the "potentiation-depotentiation"* of pallidal output.

Summary of the Dysarthria Studies. Collectively, the motor control studies of the dysarthrias in the past decade have pointed out that the perceptual-acoustic-physiologic relationships are much more complex than suggested by the initial hypotheses (Darley et al., 1969a, 1969b). Despite a certain homogeneity of perceptual dimensions for a particular type of dysarthria (e.g., parkinsonian dysarthria), a wide variety of movement and motor control problems can exist for any member of that group. Causal relationships have yet to be established between (1) given perceptual-acoustic dimensions *or* neurologic signs (flaccidity, rigidity, spasticity, etc.) *and* (2) their associated movement or motor control problems. Once such relations are fully specified, there may be as many forms of dysarthria as there are dysarthric speakers.

This is a hypothesis of challenge, rather than despair, for such specification ultimately should benefit speech remediation for the individual dysarthric subject as well as further clarify the unique aspects of human speech as a motor skill.

Only a very few dysarthric subjects have been studied with combined perceptual, acoustic, and physiologic methods. Major problems continue to exist in classifying groups or types of dysarthria by *any* criteria (e.g., perceptual, neurologic, neurophysiologic, site of lesion). Perhaps the most immediately fruitful approach will be of *case studies* with *highly restricted, well-documented* lesions to pathways or modules of the speech

---

*Following Gallistel's (1980) concept of activating complex, coordinated "units of behavior" with "direct current," or tonic, "potentiation" or "depotentiation."

motor system. Instrumentation advances allow simultaneous recording of speech movements and gEMG with adult dysarthric subjects (Barlow and Abbs, 1983). Once valid criteria are developed for identification of SMUs in the face, oropharynx, and larynx, recording of these potentials during movement (after Hannerz, 1974) should rapidly increase the understanding of speech motor control and its disorders (MacNeilage, 1973; Smith, Zimmerman, and Abbas, 1981; Sussman, MacNeilage, and Hanson, 1977).

A Physiologic Approach to a Physiologic Problem

Physiologic studies of dysarthria and dyscontrol of other motor systems have focused remediation attempts on the *functional* disabilities of the *individual* patient (cf. Grimm and Nashner, 1978; Netsell and Abbs, 1977). For example, the questions are not "Does she or he have Parkinson's disease or ataxia?" but rather "What is the disability in generating phasic muscle contractions? How are these affected by velocity or postural changes?" or "What is her or his ability to reorganize muscle forces and movements in the face of novel situations?" Physiologic answers to the latter questions form the logic of customized, physiologically based treatments of the dysarthric *individual* (Netsell and Daniel, 1979; Rosenbek and LaPointe, 1978; Rubow, 1980). These clinical developments have followed directly from the physiologic studies of normal and neurologically impaired speakers. The questions of "*What* is out of control?", "*How* is it out of control?", and "What's the optimal way to *gain* or *regain* control?" will have better answers with a better understanding of the normal and pathologic systems. These normal-abnormal comparisons also should reveal the usefulness of normal models to the study of dysarthric mechanisms and the extent to which *models of dyscontrol* may be necessary.

Developmental Dysarthrias

This selective review has focused on recent studies of *adult* dysarthrias that, in turn, have affected the thought and actions of clinicians and clients. Similar studies are needed of the normal and pathologic *development* of speech motor control. Developmental dysarthrias can be blatant, as in chronic encephalopathy (cerebral palsy), or subtle, as in neuromotor delays. Answers to questions concerning the use or misuse of (1) normal and abnormal reflexes, (2) afference, reafference, or both, and (3) neuronal pacemakers (after Gallistel, 1980) are absolutely essential to any understanding of the development of purposive speech from the purposive brain (Granit, 1977; Wolff, 1979).

POSTSCRIPT

It is my firm conviction that, in the last resort, every significant advance in neurophysiology must always refer, explicitly or implicitly, to models of how we imagine the system works, as well as to models of what we imagine the system is doing. Paying more attention to the behavioral output of the living object might teach us about the real problems to which we should direct our attention. Imagination, however, to be productive, needs to flourish on the firm ground of well established fact. That is a necessary but not sufficient condition. It needs also something else, some subtle catalyst that is provided by the interdisciplinary culture. Moreover, speculation can finally be rewarding only if it is susceptible to experiment; only then, it achieves scientific legality and the status of verifiable hypothesis.

(Paillard, 1978)

As always, the major obstacles will lie not with the sophistication of the instrumentation or data analyses, but with the quality of the experimental questions.

REFERENCES

Abbs, J., Barlow, S., and Cole, K. (1979). *Impairments of rapid muscle contraction as a physiologic feature of ataxic dysarthria.* Presented to the American Speech and Hearing Association, San Francisco.

Abbs, J., and Cole, K. (1982). Consideration of bulbar and suprabulbar afferent influences upon speech motor coordination and programming. In S. Grillner, B. Lindblom, J. Lubker, and A. Persson (Eds.), *Speech motor control* (pp. 159–186). Proceedings of an International Symposium on the Functional Basis of Oculomotor Disorders. New York: Pergamon Press.

Allen, G., and Tsukahara, N. (1974). Cerebro-cerebellar communication systems. *Physiology Reviews, 54,* 957–1006.

Barlow, S.M., and Abbs, J.H.(1983). Force transducers for the evaluation of labial, lingual, and mandibular function in dysarthria. *Journal of Speech and Hearing Research, 26,* 616–621.

Bernshtein, N. (1967). *Coordination and regulation of movements.* Oxford: Pergamon Press.

Burke, R. (1980). Motor unit types: Functional specializations in motor control. *Trends in Neuroscience, 11*(3), 255–258.

Darley, F., Aronson, A., and Brown, J. (1969a). Differential diagnostic patterns of dysarthria. *Journal of Speech and Hearing Research, 12,* 246–269.

Darley, F., Aronson, A., and Brown, J. (1969b). Clusters of deviant speech dimensions in dysarthrias. *Journal of Speech and Hearing Research, 12,* 462–496.

Darley, F., Aronson, A., and Brown, J. (1975). *Motor speech disorders.* Philadelphia: W. B. Saunders.

Desmedt, J. (Ed.) (1978). *Cerebral motor control in man: Long loop mechanisms* (Vol. 4). *Progress in clinical neurophysiology.* Basel: S. Karger.

Desmedt, J., and Godaux, E. (1978). Ballistic skilled movements: Load compensation and patterning of the motor commands. In J. E. Desmedt (Ed.), *Cerebral motor control in man: Long loop mechanisms.* Vol. 4. *Progress in clinical neurophysiology.* Basel: S. Karger.

Dubner, R., Sessle, B., and Storey, A. (1978). Peripheral components of motor control. In *The neural basis of oral and facial function.* New York: Plenum Press.

Evarts, E. (1982). Analogies between central motor programs for speech and for limb movements. In S. Grillner, B. Lindblom, J. Lubker, and A. Persson (Eds.). *Speech motor control* (pp. 19–41). Proceedings of an International Symposium on the Functional Basis of Oculomotor Disorders. New York: Pergamon Press.

Gallistel, C. (1980). From muscles to motivation. *American Scientist, 68,* 398–409.

Gay, T., Lindblom, B., and Lubker, J. (1981). Production of bite-block vowels: Acoustic equivalence by selective compensation. *Journal of the Acoustical Society of America, 69*(3), 802–810.

Gilman, S. (1969). The mechanism of cerebellar hypotonia: An experimental study in the monkey. *Brain, 92,* 621–638.

Gilman, S. (1974). A cerebello-thalamo-cortical pathway controlling fusimotor activity. In R. B. Stein, *Control of posture and locomotion.* New York: Plenum Press.

Glaser, G. (1963). Cerebellum stretch responses, and initiation of movement. In G. Walsh (Ed.), *Cerebellum, posture and cerebral palsy, Little Club Clinics in Developmental Medicine, No. 8.* London: Heinemann Medical Books Ltd.

Granit, R. (1977). *The purposive brain.* Cambridge, MA: MIT Press.

Grillner, S. (1982). Possible analogies in the control of innate motor acts and the production of sound in speech. In S. Grillner, B. Lindblom, J. Lubker, and A. Persson (Eds.), *Speech motor control* (pp. 217–229). Proceedings of an International Symposium on the Functional Basis of Oculomotor Disorders. New York: Pergamon Press.

Grimby, L., and Hannerz, J. (1974). Disturbances in the voluntary recruitment order of anterior tibial motor units in bradykinesia of parkinsonism. *Journal of Neurology, Neurosurgery, and Psychiatry, 37,* 47–54.

Grimby, L., and Hannerz, J., (1975). Disturbances in the voluntary recruitment order of anterior tibial motor units in ataxia. *Journal of Neurology, Neurosurgery, and Psychiatry, 38,* 46–51.

Grimby, L., and Hannerz, J. (1979). The afferent influence on the voluntary firing range of individual motor units in man. *Muscle and Nerve, 2,* 414–422.

Grimm, R., and Nashner, L. (1978). Long loop dyscontrol. In J. E. Desmedt (Ed.), *Cerebral motor control in man: Long loop mechanisms.* Vol. 4. *Progress in clinical neurophysiology.* Basel: S. Karger.

Gurfinkel, V., and Levik, Y. (1979). Sensory complexes and sensorimotor integration. *Fiziologiya Cheloveka, 5,* 399–414.

Hannerz, J. (1974). An electrode for recording single motor unit activity during strong muscle contractions. *Electroencephalography and Clinical Neurophysiology, 37,* 179–181.

Hardy, J. (1971). Development of neuromuscular systems underlying speech production. In *Speech and the dentofacial complex: The state of the art.* ASHA Reports, No. 5, 49–68.

Hixon, T., and Hardy, J. (1964). Restricted motility of the speech articulators in cerebral palsy. *Journal of Speech and Hearing Disorders, 29,* 293–306.

Hunker, C., Abbs, J., and Barlow, S. (1980). *Labial tonicity associated with* parkinsonian dysarthria. Paper presented to the American Speech and Hearing Association, Detroit, Michigan.

Kent, R. (1976). Anatomical and neuromuscular maturation of the speech mechanism: Evidence from acoustic studies. *Journal of Speech and Hearing Research, 19,* 422–447.

Kent, R., and Moll, K. (1975). Articulatory timing in selected consonant sequences. *Brain and Language, 2,* 304–323.

Kent, R., and Netsell, R. (1975). A case study of an ataxic dysarthric: Cinefluorographic and spectrographic observations. *Journal of Speech and Hearing Disorders, 40,* 52–71.

Kent, R., and Netsell, R. (1979). *Acoustic-phonetic features of parkinsonian dysarthria.* Paper presented to the American Speech and Hearing Association, Atlanta, Georgia.

Kent, R., Netsell, R., and Abbs, J. (1979). Acoustic characteristics of dysarthria associated with cerebellar disease. *Journal of Speech and Hearing Research, 22,* 627–648.

Kornhuber, H. (1974). Cerebral cortex, cerebellum and basal ganglia: An introduction to their motor functions. In F. Schmitt and F. Worden (Eds.), *The neurosciences: Third study program.* Cambridge, MA: MIT Press.

Kornhuber, H. (1977). A reconsideration of the cortical and subcortical mechanisms involved in speech and aphasia. In J. E. Desmedt (Ed.), *Language and hemispheric specialization in man: Event-related cerebral potentials.* Vol. 3. *Progress in clinical neurophysiology.* Basel: S. Karger.

Ladefoged, P., DeClerk, J., Lindau, M., and Papcun, G. (1972). An auditory-motor theory of speech production. *UCLA Working Papers in Phonetics,* No. 22, 48–75.

Leanderson, R., Meyerson, B., and Persson, A. (1971). The effect of L-dopa on speech in parkinsonism: An EMG study of labial articulatory function. *Journal of Neurology, Neurosurgery, and Psychiatry, 34,* 679–681.

Leanderson, R., Meyerson, B., and Persson, A. (1972). Lip muscle function in parkinsonian dysarthria. *Acta Otolaryngologica, 73,* 1–8.

Lee, R., and Tatton, W. (1978). Long loop reflexes in man: Clinical applications. In J. E. Desmedt (Ed.), *Cerebral motor control in man: Long loop mechanisms.* Vol. 4. *Progress in clinical neurophysiology.* Basel: S. Karger.

Lennerstrand, G., and Bach-y-Rita, P. (Eds.) (1975). *Basic mechanisms of ocular motility and their clinical implications.* Oxford: Pergamon Press.

Logemann, J., Fisher, H., Boshes, B., and Blonsky, E. (1978). Frequency and occurrence of vocal tract dysfunctions in the speech of a large number of Parkinson patients. *Journal of Speech and Hearing Disorders, 43,* 47–51.

Lubker, J., Kuehn, D., and Fritzell, B. (1981). Unpublished data.

MacNeilage, P. (1970). Motor control of serial ordering of speech. *Psychology Reviews, 77,* 182–196.

MacNeilage, P. (1973). Preliminaries to the study of single motor unit activity in speech musculature. *Journal of Phonetics, 1,* 55–71.

Marquardt, T. (1973). Characteristics of speech production in Parkinson's disease: Electromyographic, structural movement, and aerodynamic measurements. Doctoral dissertation, University of Washington, Seattle.

Milner-Brown, H., Stein, R., and Lee, R. (1974a). Pattern of recruiting human motor units in neuropathies and motoneuron disease. *Journal of Neurology, Neurosurgery, and Psychiatry, 37,* 665–669.

Milner-Brown, H., Stein, R., and Lee, R. (1974b). Contractile and electrical properties of human motor units in neuropathies and motoneuron disease. *Journal of Neurology, Neurosurgery, and Psychiatry, 37,* 670–675.

Milner-Brown, H., Fisher, M., and Weiner, W. (1979). Electrical properties of motor units in parkinsonism and a possible relationship with bradykinesia. *Journal of Neurology, Neurosurgery, and Psychiatry, 37,* 670–675.

Mortimer, J., and Webster, D. (1978). Relationships between quantitative measures of rigidity and tremor and the electromyographic responses to load perturbations in unselected normal subjects and Parkinson patients. In J. E. Desmedt (Ed.), *Cerebral motor control in man: Long loop mechanisms.* Vol. 4. *Progress in clinical neurophysiology.* Basel: S. Karger.

Netsell, R. (1979). Physiological bases of dysarthria. Final Report, Research Grant NS 06927, National Institutes of Health, Bethesda, MD.

Netsell, R. (1981). The acquisition of speech motor control: A perspective with directions for research. In R. Stark (Ed.), *Language behavior in infancy and early childhood* (pp. 127–153). Amsterdam: Elsevier–North Holland.

Netsell, R., and Abbs, J. (1977). Some possible uses of neuromotor speech disturbances in understanding the normal mechanism. In M. Sawashima and F. Cooper (Eds.), *Dynamic aspects of speech production.* Tokyo: University of Tokyo Press.

Netsell, R., and Daniel, B. (1979). Dysarthria in adults. *Archives of Physical Medicine and Rehabilitation, 60,* 502–508.

Netsell, R., Daniel, B., and Celesia, G. (1975). Acceleration and weakness in parkinsonian dysarthria. *Journal of Speech and Hearing Disorders, 40,* 170–178.

Netsell, R., and Kent, R. (1976). Paroxysmal ataxic dysarthria. *Journal of Speech and Hearing Disorders, 41,* 93–109.

Netsell, R., Kent, R., and Abbs, J. (1980). The organization and reorganization of speech movements. Presented at Society for Neuroscience, Cincinnati, OH.

Ojemann, G., and Mateer, K. (1980). Human language cortex: Localization of memory, syntax, and sequential motor phoneme identification systems. *Science, 205,* 1401–1403.

Paillard, J. (1978). The pyramidal tract: Two million fibres in search of a function. *Journal de Physiologie, 74,* 155–162.

Persson, A. (Ed.) (1979). Proceedings of the 6th International Congress of Electromyography. *Acta Neurological Scandinavica, 60,* Suppl. 73.

Petajan, J., and Jarcho, L. (1975). Motor unit control in Parkinson's disease and the influence of levodopa. *Neurology, 25,* 866–869.

Ploog, D. (1979). Phonation, emotion, cognition, with reference to the brain mechanisms involved. In *Brain and Mind,* CIBA Foundation Symposium, No. 69. Amsterdam: Elsevier–North Holland.

Quaglieri, C., and Celesia, G. (1977). Effect of thalamotomy and levodopa therapy on the speech of Parkinson patients. *European Neurology, 15,* 34–39.

Robinson, B. (1976). Limbic influences on human speech. *Annals of the New York Academy of Science, 280,* 761–771.

Rosenbek, J., and LaPointe, L. (1978). The dysarthrias: Description, diagnosis and treatment. In D. Johns (Ed.), *Clinical management of neurogenic communicative disorders.* Boston: Little, Brown and Co.

Rubow, R. (1980). Biofeedback treatment of speech disorders. In *Biofeedback Society of America Task Force Reports.* Wheat Ridge, CO.

Scheibel, A. (1979). Development of axonal and dendritic neuropil as a function of evolving behavior. In F. Schmitt and F. Worden (Eds.), *The neurosciences fourth study program.* Cambridge, MA: MIT Press.

Scott, A. (1975). Strabismus-muscle forces and innervations. In G. Lennerstrand

and P. Bach-y-Rita (Eds.), *Basic mechanisms of ocular motility and their clinical implications*. New York: Pergamon Press.

Smith, A., Zimmerman, G., and Abbas, P. (1981). Recruitment patterns of motor units in speech production. *Journal of Speech and Hearing Research, 24,* 567–576.

Steklis, H., and Raleigh, M. (1979). Requisites for language: Interspecific and evolutionary aspects. In H. Steklis and M. Raleigh (Eds.), *Neurobiology of social communication in primates*. New York: Academic Press.

Studdert-Kennedy, M. (1980). The beginnings of speech. In G. Barlow, K. Immelmann, M. Main, and L. Petrinovich (Eds.), *Behavioral development: The Bielefeld interdisciplinary project*. New York: Cambridge University Press.

Sussman, H., MacNeilage, P., and Hanson, R. (1977). Recruitment and discharge patterns of single motor units during speech production. *Journal of Speech and Hearing Research, 20,* 613–630.

Sutton, D., Larson, C., and Lindeman, R. (1974). Neocortical and limbic lesion effects on primate phonation. *Brain Research, 71,* 61–75.

Terzuolo, C., and Viviani, P. (1974). Movements, parameters and EMG activities during some simple motor tasks in normal subjects and cerebellar patients. In I.S. Cooper, M. Riklan, and R. Snider (Eds.), *Cerebellum, epilepsy and behavior*. Oxford: Pergamon Press.

Vignon, C., Pellissier, J., and Serratrice, G. (1980). Further histochemical studies on masticatory muscles. *Journal of Neurological Sciences, 45,* 157–176.

Watkin, K., and Fromm, D. (19xx). Development of labial coordination in children during the production of selected speech stimuli.

White, N., and Kinesbourne, M. (1980). Does speech output control lateralize over time? Evidence from verbal-manual time-sharing tasks. *Brain and Language, 10,* 215–223.

Wolff, P. (1979). *Theoretical issues in the development of motor skills*. Symposium on Developmental Disabilities in the Pre-School Child, Johnson & Johnson Baby Products, Chicago, IL.

Chapter 3

A Neurobiologic View of the Dysarthrias

PROLOGUE

A Definition of Dysarthria

This chapter emphasizes a neurobiologic view of individuals whose speech is considered to be dysarthric. Dysarthria is defined here as a *speech* disorder resulting from damage to *neural mechanisms* that *regulate* speech movements. The word "speech" in this definition is intended to distinguish dysarthria from language disorders (aphasias) or more broadly based cognitive disorders. The use of "regulate" in the definition serves to distinguish dysarthria from apraxia of speech, in which the latter results from damage to neural mechanisms responsible for selecting, sequencing, and (perhaps) constructing the spatial-temporal goals of a given speech act.

A Neurobiologic View

In this chapter, a neurobiologic view is developed that emphasizes evolutionary and biologic determinants of speech and its neurologic dis-

Reprinted by permission of the publisher from *The dysarthrias: Physiology, acoustics, perception, management*, M. McNeil, J. Rosenbek, and A. Aronson (Eds.), pp. 1–36. Copyright 1984 by College-Hill Press, Inc., San Diego, California.

orders. Optimal treatment of an individual with dysarthria represents the best fitting of available treatment procedures to our best *understanding* of the determinants of that individual's speech patterns. In seeking such an understanding, a neurobiologic approach emphasizes the "interactionist model" of physiologic and external environmental variables (after Wolff, 1981).

> The "interactionist model" offers a viable alternative to either of the extreme formulations, because it can integrate data on both physiological (genetic, hormonal, neurological) and experiential determinants without a commitment to either factor as a sufficient cause. . . . Physiologic processes prepare the organism to respond appropriately to environmental events that will promote its psychological and physiological development. Experience has potent physiological and structure effects, as well as behavioral consequences. Therefore, the causal chain is as likely to proceed from experience to physiology and structure formation as from structure to behavior.
>
> (Wolff, 1981, p. 1)

The neurobiologic view presented here is that the current status of the human nervous system can best be understood against the background of (1) its evolution, including that of nonhuman primates (i.e., phylogeny), (2) the development of the individual's nervous system, as influenced by its phylogeny and interactions with its environment (i.e., ontogeny), and (3) the "survival value" of the behaviors of interest (in particular, the vocal expressions of emotion and thought). These three areas represent the basic tenets of ethology, a discipline that Tinbergen (1963) stated was basically the study of the biology of behavior.

An Underlying Premise

The premise underlying the search for a better understanding of the dysarthrias is that this knowledge will benefit individuals with the problem, as well as those who may suffer brain injury in the future. Whereas even 20 to 25 years ago there was little evidence that treatment could be a major influence in recovery from brain injury, current thinking and data reflect a considerable optimism (cf. Bach-y-Rita, 1980; Finger and Stein, 1982). Another benefit of studying speech and neurologic conditions from a neurobiologic perspective should be an increase in our understanding of the origins, extant behaviors, and future behaviors of human communication (in particular) and the hominid (in general). Two articles illustrate the above statements. Brodal (1973), a neuroanatomist, provided insightful neurophysiologic hypotheses about the differential effects of spontaneous recovery and various therapies, based on self-observations following a stroke. Pribram (1982), in developing thoughts for a "neurobiologic theory of music," draws striking parallels to human language.

A Review of Reviews

Given some obvious limitations (including page allocation and the opinions of the author), this chapter necessarily represents a "review of reviews" in that many of the references cited are summaries of large bodies of information. As with any review, this one is selective and oversights in referencing as well as inaccuracies in interpretation are inevitable. To those who will feel slighted or misunderstood, I sympathize in advance.

The plan for this chapter is to (1) provide a historical perspective for the emergence of dysarthria as a topic for interdisciplinary study, (2) summarize more recent advances in understanding the nervous system, speech motor control, and neuropathophysiology, and (3) relate these issues to the treatment of dysarthria.

HISTORICAL DEVELOPMENTS

A neurobiologic view of the dysarthrias has roots traceable to individuals and groups who emphasized speech physiology, its evolutionary development, or both. This historical perspective pertains basically to those developments in the twentieth century and in the United States. What seems clear is that parallel approaches were being developed in the United States and Soviet Union, and recent translations of Luria (1970, 1981) reveal the strong influence of the "interactionist model" in the Russians' view of human communication and its disorders. Indeed, by the definitions given above, the work of Pavlov, Bechterew, Schenkov, Anokhin, Bernshtein, and Vygotsky was embodied by Luria in a truly neurobiologic sense. Luria emphasized a "functional systems" analysis of cognition-language-speech disorders, anticipating or paralleling, as always, the directions and development of other researchers.

1900–1950

The start of the period 1900–1950 seems most clearly marked to me by the dissertation of John Muyskens (1925) at the University of Michigan titled *The Hypha*. The hypha was regarded as a "physiological syllable" and represents a clear forerunner of the continuing search for "basic units" of speech production. One of Muyskens's students, Shohara, made one of the earliest and clearest statements about "coarticulatory effects" in her 1932 dissertation titled *Genesis of Articulatory Movements of Speech* (see also Shohara, 1939). Two of Muyskens's other doctoral students, Westlake and Palmer, were major influences in examining and treating speech disorders of children with cerebral palsy. These individuals and their students strongly advocated a position that "speech was an overlaid function," a point to be discussed later in this chapter. The foundations for this point of view were in completed manuscript form by 1938, but publication was delayed until after World War II (Meader and Muyskens, 1950).

The arrival of Froschels in this country in the mid to late 1930s also had great impact on this period's research and treatment of the dysarthrias, including adult dysarthrias. Froschels's view also was clearly neurobiologic, if you will, as evidenced in the English translation of his 1918 monograph *Childhood Language and Aphasia* (Rieber, 1980). Consider, as examples, the following chapter titles: "Reflections on the history of evolution of speech and the faults of an evolutionary approach," "The first stage of speech: Crying," "Babbling: The emergence of sensory components of the speech mechanism," and "The path from thinking to speaking."

The research of Stetson in this period also was a clear antecedent to present work on the motor control of speech and limb movements (Stetson, 1950). The work of Stetson and his colleagues, as well as Muyskens, formed the bases for biologic views of speech production in the literature for the first half of the twentieth century.

1950–1970

The quantitative research in the years 1950–1970 emphasized differences between normal *group* performance and that of selected dysarthric subgroups. Examples included studies of parkinsonian dysarthria (cf. Canter, 1963, 1965a, 1965b) and children with cerebral palsy (Hardy, 1964). For the most part, university coursework covered the dysarthrias in children (e.g., cerebral palsy) and adults (as part of "Adult Neuropathologies of Speech and Language") in separate classes, and many students may have missed the phylo-ontogenetic information of the former and the speech physiology data of the latter.

During this period, Lenneberg (with *Biological Foundations of Language*, 1967) carried on the Muyskens tradition of accounting for evolutionary and biologic influences on the ontogeny of speech-language development and its disorders.

What seems clear to me from this short history is that the call for physiologic research of the dysarthrias near the end of this period (Darley, Aronson, and Brown, 1969a, 1969b; Hardy, 1966) was a logical extension of the preceding 50 years.

The 1970s

Research on dysarthria early in the 1970s was marked by physiologic studies of the moment to moment changes in muscle contractions and vocal tract movements (e.g., Kent, 1973; Logemann, Fisher, Boshes, and Blonsky, 1978; Netsell, 1971). Even these largely qualitative studies came rapidly to influence the clinical procedures of evaluation and treatment of individual dysarthric clients (e.g., Darley, Aronson, and Brown, 1975; Netsell and Daniel, 1979; Rosenbek and LaPointe, 1978; Rubow, 1980). The establishment of an NIH Clinical Research Center at the University of Wisconsin in 1977 brought together an interdisciplinary team of basic and clinical scientists to study neurogenic speech disorders. That work incorporates a combined systems analysis and a neurophysiologic approach to these problems and those studies are responsible, in large part, for the marked increase in our current understanding of the dysarthrias (e.g., Abbs, Hunker, and Barlow, 1983; Abbs and Kennedy, 1980; Barlow and Abbs, 1984; Hunker and Abbs, 1984; Hunker, Abbs, and Barlow, 1982; Müller, Abbs, and Kennedy, 1981).

This physiologic research of the 1970s was almost entirely with adult dysarthrics and normal adult controls. Comparable studies of children with dysarthria are a clear research need, as will be elaborated below.

UNDERSTANDING THE DYSARTHRIAS

This section contains three major parts: understanding the (1) nervous system, (2) speech motor control, and (3) neuropathology. The intent is to show that this collective knowledge will enhance our understanding overall for individuals with dysarthria and optimal ways in which to treat their particular problems in gaining or regaining the ability to produce intelligible speech.

Understanding the Nervous System

Most clinical speech examinations represent a "time slice" view of the individual's speech patterns, with inferences to the underlying neuropathology. The review in this section emphasizes the continuously *evolving* nature of the nervous system, with special reference to the *distributed* and *interactive* neural mechanisms of speech and other behavior. Attention also is drawn to new data in neurotransmitter research and their relevance to understanding motor development in normal and disordered nervous systems.

Phylogeny

The study of phylogeny permits formulation of hypotheses based on the comparison of human evolution of brain-behavior characteristics with those of other animals. In comparing human and nonhuman primate vocalizations, it is assumed that there are neurobiologic and behavioral homologues, with the human advances representing a further differentiation and elaboration of the more primitive forms.

The current human nervous system has been depicted as a composite of reticular, limbic, and neocortical systems (MacLean, 1970; Moore, 1980; Mysak, 1976). The phylogenetically older parts (reticular and limbic) sufficed once to meet the survival needs of the organism, including communication, remaining with us to serve basic biologic responses (e.g., homeostasis, equilibrium, postural reactions, and feeding) and "affective-emotional" communications, including crying, laughing, and facial expressions.

The neocortical system has evolved for expression of finer sensorimotor skills, including speech, music, and perhaps thought as well (Luria, 1981). The superior analytic skills (sensory, cognitive, and motor) of the human also are attributed to neocortical developments. The term "cortical" in "neocortical" can give the false impression that the "higher cortical functions" of humans have their anatomic focus in the cerebral cortex. As described later, the neocortical system is distributed throughout the subcortical anatomy, including in the cerebellum. This helps explain why subcortical lesions in humans can have analytic as well as affective-emotional consequences for communication disorders (Brown, 1979; Kent, 1984).

In considering the human communication lessons to be learned from nonhuman primates, it is most advantageous when the latter have vocalizations in their repertoire that are "intentional" as well as "affective," in which the former might be regarded as antecedents of human "analytic" speech. Even when this distinction is not clear, as for example in the squirrel monkey, the implications are provocative (cf. Jurgens, 1979; Ploog, 1979, 1981). The squirrel monkey has a hierarchical organization of vocal control. At the top of this hierarchy is the cortex around the anterior cingulate cortex. This area seems to be responsible for the volitional initiation of phonation. The area's most important projections are those to the sensorimotor face cortex and to the periaqueductal region in the caudal midbrain. The face cortex, presumably responsible for the motor control of learned phonatory patterns, also projects to the periaqueduct but has other pathways to brainstem nuclei. Motivational, or innate, vocalizations survive lesions at higher centers and the cingulate region seems to exert only a facilitative or inhibitory influence on these calls. On the other hand, cingulate lesions disrupt the initiation of learned vocalization and face cortex lesions affect the motor coordination of these sound productions. These results point to separate pathways for the expression of innate and learned vocalizations and will be related inferentially to human vocalizations in the section entitled *Understanding Neuropathology* later in this chapter.

For a recent review of possible hemispheric differences in the organization of speech production, see Kent (1984). P. MacNeilage (personal communication, 1983) is developing the hypothesis that the motor control for speech has evolved from the neural mechanisms used for bimanual coordination. The notion is that humans first developed bimanual coordination by holding objects in the left hand and working on or manipulating them with the right hand. MacNeilage further reasons that rather than trying to control each hand separately from the contralateral hemisphere, our ancestors developed control of bimanual coordination through one hemisphere, that is, the left. As a later development, we used many of these left brain neuronal connectivities (or similar homologues) for the motor control of speech.

Ontogeny

The ontogeny of human infant vocalization proceeds from the early innate expressions of need to those of "intended," learned vocalizations of *words* toward the end of their first year of life. The ontogeny of early word vocalizations is a subject of current research, as is the continuity-discontinuity issue of their origins in babbling and imitation (e.g., Bauer, Kent, and Murray 1983; Oller, 1981). Neural maturation and vocal tract morphology undergo continuous changes through infancy and early childhood and parallel closely the motoric complexity of the developing vocalizations (see Chapter 1 and Kent, 1981). Neural maturation also progresses from brainstem to cortical regions in this period and, given the earlier discussion of phylogeny and separate pathways for innate and learned vocalizations, the natural history of speech motor development shows ontogeny to recapitulate phylogeny—at least in this regard.

The ontogeny of speech also qualifies speech production as a motor skill (see Chapter 1 and Wolff, 1979). It seems impossible, if not unnecessary, at this point to differentiate the development of speech motor skill from related skill development (e.g., sensory, perceptual, and cognitive). If, as Luria (1981) contends, speech development in some way shapes cognitive development, any distinction may be arbitrary. Regardless, delays in speech motor development may be related more to "learning disabilities" than has been apparent to date.

A tenet of ethology is that most behaviors have a survival value, whereby the supporting anatomy and physiology have undergone and continue to undergo a continuous adaptation and further differentiation (Tinbergen, 1963). Vocalization, as a motor skill and expression of cognition language, has evolved as a survival mechanism (communication), as a means of social interaction, and as a facilitator of thought. The vocalization reflects both the emotional and analytic state of the animal, in that both speech and music contain this interaction in humans and express our most differentiated thoughts. Human "survival" and evolution obviously depend on the quality of these expressions.

The Role of Neurotransmitters

There have been several recent and major advances in understanding the contribution of neurotransmitters to mood, cognition, and activity (see reviews of Coyle, 1983; Johnston and Coyle, 1981).

> Inter-neuronal communication is mediated primarily by chemical neurotransmitters, which are released from the nerve terminal, diffuse across the synaptic cleft and interact with specific receptors on adjacent neurons. The development of the biochemical machinery for neurotransmission is closely linked to the functional maturation of the brain's neuronal circuitry. Components essential for neurotransmission (e.g., synthetic enzymes, endogenous neurotransmitters, re-uptake processes and receptors) serve as specific biochemical markers for neuronal systems. The appearance of and developmental increases in these markers during fetal and postnatal life occur with the cessation of neuronal replication and initiation of neuropil elaboration. Discrete groups of neurotransmitter-specific neurons develop according to different timetables, resulting in a shifting pattern of their relative influence in the maturing brain.
>
> (Johnston and Coyle, 1981, p. 251)

Coyle (1983) emphasized four discrete neuronal groups, with differing loci in the nervous system, specific and often overlapping terminations, and different developmental courses. Also described are their differential effects on mood, cognition, and activity. Concerning the developmental course of these neurotransmitters, Coyle adds:

> The noradrenergic pathways appear to be among the first to develop and their axons invade cerebral cortex during the very process of its formation. Thus, the noradrenergic input would appear to be an early and consistent source of innervation to the cerebral cortex and limbic systems. The serontonergic neurons develop somewhat later and appear to provide a more gradual developmental elaboration of their processes with the cortex and limbic system. The dopaminergic neurons exhibit a somewhat delayed innervation of the cortical limbic system and with the nigrostriatal dopaminergic projection appear to exhibit a gradual and progressive innervation over the first decade and one-half of postnatal life. Finally, the cholinergic projections to cerebral cortex develop in a delayed but rather abrupt fashion. This appears to occur during the first year of life in the human.
>
> (Coyle, 1983, p. 2)

In general, the neurotransmitters provide a facilitative or suppressive effect on interneuronal communications, and these effects indirectly influence mood, cognition, and motor activity. With additional neurotransmitter research, we should better understand their influence on the development of speech motor control and its relationship to cognition as expressed through language. For example, Coyle (1983) mentioned that if autistic children do develop language, they do so around ages 4 to 5, a time when serotonin is known to sharply increase in the brain. Interestingly, this is a time when normal children rapidly increase the motoric complexity of their speech.

Further advances in understanding the developmental course and behavioral influences of each neurotransmitter should markedly influence our concepts of neuronal development and its contributions to emerging normal and pathologic behavior. Even the modest beginnings in this area have guided neurologists in pharmacologic treatments (see reviews in Ferrendelli, 1983; Rosenberg, 1983).

Understanding the Motor Control of Speech

Recent developments in our understanding of normal speech motor control have made an immediate impact on our ability to evaluate and

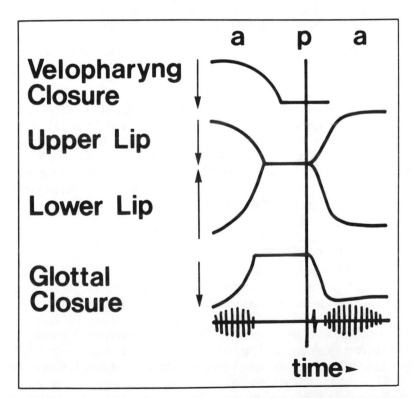

Figure 3-1. A schematic representation of the coordination of four structures in reaching a *spatial-temporal* goal. See text for discussion.

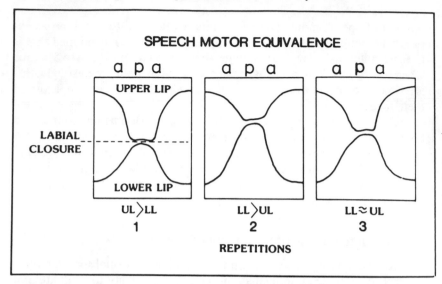

Figure 3–2. Upper and lower lip movements for three repetitions of the syllables [apa]. Repetition 1: Upper lip movement greater than lower lip. Repetition 2: Lower lip movement greater than upper lip. Repetition 3: Equal contributions of upper and lower lip movement. From Abbs, J. H., and Rosenbek, J. C. (1985). Some motor control perspectives on apraxia of speech and dysarthria. In J. Costello (Ed.), *Speech Disorders in Adults* (pp. 22–57). San Diego: College-Hill Press.

treat the dysarthrias (e.g., see Chapter 4 in this book and Abbs et al., 1983; Rosenbek and LaPointe, 1978: Yorkston and Beukelman, 1981). As indicated previously, major advances have occurred in this area in the past decade (see review in Abbs and Cole, 1982). Earlier controversy regarding the (1) playing out of "overlearned" motor patterns versus (2) the use of peripheral afference to guide speech movements during their execution has resolved to some intermediate position.

Normal Adult Performance

Spatial-Temporal Goals. In attempting to generate the meaningful acoustics of speech, the speaker must bring the vocal tract to rather precise shapes at rather precise points in time. Figure 3–1 depicts one such *spatial-temporal goal* (see Chapter 1 and Grillner, 1982; Lubker, 1982). In producing the syllable [pa], a reasonably tight velopharyngeal closure must occur before lip release, and the glottis must be open before the lip release. This spatial-temporal precision occurs roughly in the time frame of 100 ms. Since the [p] production places no requirements on the tongue, this structure already positioned (or is moving into position) for the [ɑ] sound. This is one example of movements overlapping one another, in

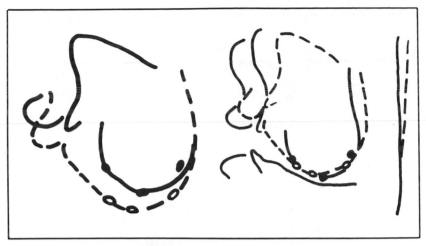

Figure 3–3. Midsagittal line drawings of upper airways for [i] vowel productions. *Left side:* Superimpositions of lip, tongue, pharynx, and jaw positions when the jaw was free to move (solid lines) and when it was held in a fixed position (dashed lines). *Right side:* Superimpositions of tongue shapes referenced to the jaw that show the extent of adjustment made with the tongue to achieve the tongue positions on the left.

which one spatial-temporal goal is being achieved as another is being formed. This also is an example of the popular term "coarticulation." (See Hammarberg, 1982, for a thorough discussion of coarticulation.) Note also that for the production of [ɑ] the glottis must move rapidly from opening on the [p] to closing for the voicing of [ɑ].

Motor Equivalence. Motor equivalence refers to the achievement of the same spatial-temporal goal throughout a variety of motor acts. In the example given earlier, the initial goal was to achieve lip closure for the [p] sound. Figure 3–2 shows that successive attainments of this goal are achieved by a variety of upper lip, lower lip, and jaw movements.

In achieving the vocal tract shape for [i], it appears necessary to reach only an "acoustically critical configuration" in the anterior oral cavity. Figure 3–3 compares the tongue shape for [i] when the jaw was free to move (solid lines) with its shape when the subject held a bite-block between the teeth, resulting in a fixed distance of 16 mm between the upper and lower incisors. With the bite-block in place, the tongue automatically reached the [i] goal, i.e., the speaker made these adjustments without any "conscious" effort to do so. Perkell and Nelson (1982) suggest that because most English vowels require quite distinct vocal tract shapes, tongue positioning for repeated productions of the same vowel can vary by a few millimeters and still generate the requisite acoustics. Thus, whereas the bite-block studies reveal the precision of which we are capable, the precision used in conversational speech can be much less.

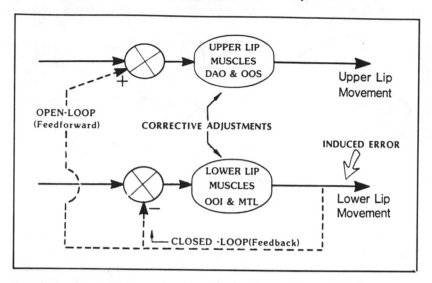

Figure 3–4. Schematic drawing to illustrate closed-loop (feedback) and open-loop (feedforward) mechanisms to the lips. See text for discussion. From Abbs, J. H., and Gracco, V. L. (1984). Control of complex motor gestures: Orofacial muscle responses to load perturbations of the lip during speech. *Journal of Neurophysiology, 51,* 705–723.

Given these examples of motor equivalence, it seems that the nervous system initially specifies the "goals" and leaves the details to be worked out—based, in part, on knowledge of the instantaneous state of the vocal 0tract. (See further discussion in Abbs and Kennedy, 1980.) How this might be accomplished is discussed in the next section.

Afferent Influences. Consideration of afferent influences incorporates the concepts of "feedback" and "feedforward" (see Abbs and Cole, 1982; Evarts, 1982). These concepts are depicted in Figure 3–4. The *feedback* system is involved whenever information about the muscle action and movement is returned directly to the neural components regulating that action. *Feedforward* is used when information regarding the peripheral state is used to alter movements of other structures in order to achieve the particular spatial-temporal goal. In Figure 3–4, the feedback from the lower lip may be used in regulating its movement for the bilabial contact, while the same information is fed forward to be used in adjustments of the upper lip to effect the contact. Presumably, mechanisms such as these are operating in the trade-offs (motor equivalence) of the lips, as shown in Figure 3–3. Abbs and Cole (1982) hypothesize the feedback system to be useful in regulating movements within 100 ms of the final goal achievement, whereas the "feedforward" feature permits adjustments to be made up until 50 ms of goal achievement. Grillner (1982) speculates

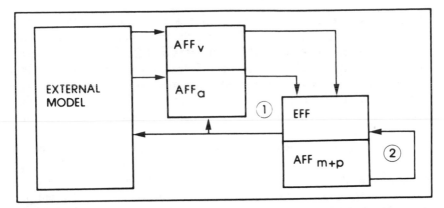

Figure 3-5. A block diagram of elements hypothesized to function in the acquisition of speech motor control. See text for discussion. From Netsell, R. (1981). The acquisition of speech motor control: A perspective with directions for research. In R. Stark (Ed.), *Language behavior in infancy and early childhood*. New York: Elsevier-North Holland. Reprinted with permission.

that information from any relevant receptor system that is available may be utilized *at the time* a movement is planned to "construct" the motor command to be issued, so as to achieve an optimal pattern of activity. With this concept, there is essentially instantaneous appraisal of the motoneurons generating the muscle forces concerning the state of the vocal tract. Earlier concerns that nervous system delays were too long for such fast modulations of motoneuron activity have been lessened by more recent theory and data (Abbs and Cole, 1982; Cole, 1981).

Learning to Talk. Little is known about the physiologic processes developed and used by normal children in learning the motor skills of speech. Knowledge of these processes is critical to understanding the dysarthrias of children (see reviews in Chapters 1 and 4 of this book.)

Afferent or Efferent Processes. Figure 3-5 is a block diagram of afferent and efferent processes that have been hypothesized to operate as the infant or child is learning to talk. These ideas have been expressed elsewhere, including in Chapter 1 and in Hardy (1970), Meader and Muyskens (1950), and Rutherford (1967). It is hypothesized that the normal child learns to talk by listening, watching, and imitating an external model (e.g., a parent, caregiver, or other child). The model provides both auditory and visual afferent cues (AFF[a] and AAF[v]) which the child attempts to imitate with his or her own movements and vocalizations (shown as EFF, efferent). This EFF has two important consequences. First, it generates the auditory patterns that return to the ears of the model and child. The latter auditory feedback closes the important motor-auditory loop shown as (1) in Figure 3–5. Second EEF creates feedback associated with the speech movements and postures (AAF^{m+p}) that the child pairs with his or her auditory patterns. In essence, the child hears and feels his or her speech movements as they are being developed. This tight sensorimotor-auditory coupling presumably is the key to his refinement of the output (EFF) to approximate the external model. By this process, the child eventually develops internal representations in his or her nervous system of these sensorimotor activities.

It is not clear at this point that the child uses conscious control of speech movements in learning to talk. He or she may unconsciously develop control of speech movements in a manner similar to the way that adults unconsciously generate their speech movements. Intervention strategies that bring speech movement routines to a level of visual or kinesthetic awareness may be contrary to these more natural control processes (see discussion in Chapter 4). Future behavioral interventions will benefit from research that clarifies the manner in which speech motor control is learned.

From Phonology to Physiology. The naturalness of fundamental phonetic units (e.g., syllables of CV, VC, and VCV shape) may best be viewed as physiologic artifacts of the infant's speech-motor capability. The speech motor capability of the infant in the first 12 months is influenced most strongly by the status of his or her neural maturation and musculoskeletal system development. Similar physiologic influences on phonologic development should be sought for second explanations of language development in the second year of life. As stated by Peterson and Shoup (1966), "There is considerable reason to believe that the phonologic aspects of speech are primarily organized in terms of the possibilities and constraints of the motor mechanism with which speech is produced" (p. 7).

Distributed Systems and Functions

Another important concept is that of *distributed* systems, especially in the neocortical system (Mountcastle, 1978) (Fig. 3–6). The concept here is that nuclei in different regions of the nervous system form interconnections to serve particular functions. Some functions share particular nuclei and pathways and not others. In addition, the "command neurons" for the different functions are located at different places in the nervous system. For example, breathing, sucking, chewing, and swallowing are thought to be driven by pacemaker neurons, or pattern generators, located in the brainstem, whereas human speech motor control depends on more recently evolved neocortical structures.

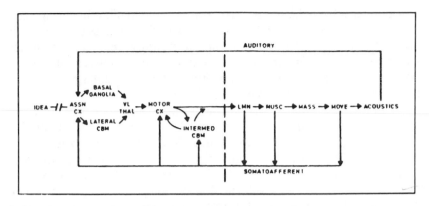

Figure 3-6. Diagrammatic representation of neural pathways, modules, and the musculoskeletal system hypothesized to be used in the motor control of speech. See text for discussion. From Netsell, R. (1982). Speech control and selected neurologic disorders. In S. Grillner, B. Lindblom, J. Lubker, and A. Persson (Eds.), *Speech motor control*. New York: Pergamon Press. Reprinted with permission.

UNDERSTANDING NEUROPATHOLOGY

In this section, an attempt is made to relate the previous discussions to neuropathology in the human nervous system, with particular reference to the neural mechanisms involved in the dysarthrias. Clearly, all that is written here is speculative, and as such, it forms only the most rudimentary hypotheses for elaboration and experimental study.

Evolving and Interactive Systems

Reticular, Limbic and Neocortical Systems

Even though an earlier distinction was made between reticular, limbic, and neocortical systems, lesions often affect more than one of these. These systems are evolutionary in a phylogenetic and maturational sense; also, they are interactive and distributed throughout the nervous system in an anatomic and functional sense.

The reticular system, extending from lower to higher brainstem and including the basal nuclei, is both diffuse and specific in its organization and function. Lesions to respiratory centers, of course, are not compatible with life. Lesser lesions result in postural reactions (e.g., asymmetric tonic neck reflexes, righting reactions) that obligate the muscles and body parts to rather fixed postures and impair attempts at fine muscle contractions (Moore, 1980; Mysak, 1976, 1980). Patients with these problems reportedly gain relief from the symptoms through manipulations in the high cervical regions (cf. Moore, 1980; Mysak, 1980). The reticular system also is believed to be "sensory oriented," in that multiple and specific sensory inputs collect there. One therapy rationale is aimed at differential stimulation of these sensory channels via peripheral nerves of differing diameter. (See discussions of M. Rood in Harris, 1969, 1971.)

Damage to the limbic system affects the individual's control of affect and the initiation of movement (Brown, 1979; Kent, 1984). Uncontrolled bouts of crying or laughing often occur, as do vocalizations of a guttural or banal nature. What seems to be lacking is the engagement of the neocortical system for the purposes of "ideational" speech. More severe involvement of limbic structures results in akinetic mutism (Brown, 1979; Kent, 1984). Recalling Ploog's work (1981) with squirrel monkeys discussed previously, lesions to the cingulate cortex left them unable to carry out "learned vocalizations," whereas their "affective" calls survived. Even neurologically normal speakers can have their speech nearly halted during moments of extreme anxiety. It is tempting to speculate that neurochemical thresholds in the limbic system can fluctuate, and, indeed, are more labile in certain neuropathologic conditions of the limbic system as well as during the more emotional movements of normal individuals.

The neocortical system, as the phylogenetically most advanced and maturationally last to develop, is believed responsible for all the human's most highly differentiated behaviors (including sensory, perceptual, motor, and cognitive). Cortical damage to the neocortical system (see Fig. 3–6) can be massive outside of Broca's, Wernicke's, and the supplementary motor areas—with intelligible speech preserved (Finger and Stein, 1982; Penfield and Roberts, 1959). Much smaller lesions at "summing points" for multiple inputs (e.g., Broca's area, motor sensory cortex, or cerebellum) can result in a dyspraxia or dysarthria. Brodal (1973), for example, believed his lesion was restricted to the right internal capsule and he reported problems with fine motor control of speech and writing that included errors of an apraxic nature, as well as dysarthria. This raises the issue as to whether or not apraxia of speech and dysarthria can appear separately when the neocortical system is damaged. Certainly, many apraxic speakers sound ataxic, and the converse. Considering also that apraxic subjects have problems in constructing individual spatial-temporal goals (see Fig. 3–1) as well as the serial ordering of those goals (see Fromm, 1981), the dyspraxic-dysarthric distinction becomes less clear in the neocortical system. The following discussion of evolving anterior and posterior systems may help to clarify some of the shared versus specialized systems for speech processes that, when impaired, yield symptoms we classify as dysarthric and dyspraxic, respectively.

Anterior Versus Posterior Systems

Several authors, including Brown (1979), Mysak (1980), and Penfield and Roberts (1959), point to neuroanatomic and physiologic distinctions between an *anterior* and *posterior* system development that predominantly serve the production and perception components of speech, respectively. Brown reviews literature to support his view that anterior system damage results in several forms of expressive aphasia. He also points to the evolutionary and maturational progression of these systems through the reticular-to-limbic-to-neocortical developments, with the forms of speech-language disturbance falling on a continuum from "old brain" to "new brain." Brown (1979) also introduces the concept of an evolving "motor envelope."

> The developing utterance issues out of a preliminary (limbic) cognition. Simultaneously, the action of the limbs proceeds outward towards objects in extrapersonal space. The diffuse, labile affect of the limbic level is derived into more differentiated partial expressions while consciousness of speech and action becomes increasingly more critical and acute.
>
> From the point of view of the speech act, there is a progression from akinetic mutism, an inability to evoke or further realize the motor envelope of the speech act, through an attenuated form of transcortical motor aphasia, to agrammatism and finally Broca's aphasia proper. In this progression, the cognitive stage, as it is revealed in pathology, becomes increasingly more focused as it develops toward the final articulatory units.
>
> The motor envelope contains the embryonic speech act together with its accompanying gestural and somatic motor elements. At this stage, the elements are only prefigurative, bearing little resemblance to the performance (speech, gesture) to which they give rise.
>
> At the point where the speech act differentiates out of this background organization, pathological disruption is characterized by a lack of spontaneous or conversational speech with good repetition. At times, naming and reading aloud are also spared. This constellation of findings has been termed *transcortical motor aphasia*; it is similar to the dynamic aphasia of Luria. In this syndrome, there is more than just a lack of spontaneous speech; nonspeech vocalizations and gestures are also reduced and there is often an inertia of the behavior generally, which may suggest parkinsonism. These "associated" symptoms all point to a common level or origin in the unfolding motor act; they are also a sign of its proximity to akinetic mutism.
>
> This disorder reflects an involvement at the level of generation of an utterance, a speech act, without a disruption of the (potential) constituents of that act. This may concern the initiation of the utterance, its organization, and/or its differentiation from other motor elements at that level. Repetition aids in achieving this differentiation and in providing a configuration through which syntactic differentiation can occur. Naming is frequently preserved. The presence of an object may help to provide a structure through which this differentiation may occur. The presence of good naming in this disorder marks a transition to the next level, that of agrammatism, where

there is also superior noun production.

The affective state of such patients is usually one of apathy or indifference. The apparent lack of emotional responsiveness is another feature indicating a link with cingulate gyrus disorders. However, the pathological anatomy is uncertain. At least it can be said that the preservation of repetition is not to be understood by the sparing of a repetition pathway; that is, it is not a transcortical defect (Brown, 1975). In many cases there is partial involvement of the left Broca area (Goldstein, 1915). I have described a case with subtotal destruction of Broca's area (Brown, 1975). On the other hand, the most frequent cause is probably occlusion of the anterior cerebral artery, which entails damage to the anterior cingulate gyrus, supplementary motor area and contiguous structures on the medial surface of the frontal lobe. Conceivably, the disorder may follow a left cingulate lesion as a partial form of the severe mutism with bilateral cingulate destruction. The association with supplementary motor area is now well-established. These contain limbic-derived neocortical zones. In any event, the correlation is either with limbic-transitional or *meso*cortex or with the next level in neocortical phylogenesis, generalized neocortex of the left frontal region.

As the speech act differentiates, the simpler and more global units of the utterance-to-be are the first to emerge. Along with the appearance of nouns and uninflected verbs, there is an unfolding into the forming utterance of the small grammatical or function words. The appearance of the functors is thus delayed to a level of individuation subsequent to that of holophrastic noun and verb production. Disorders at this stage are characterized by an incomplete differentiation of emerging syntactic units (agrammatism).

Conceivably, this disturbance can be conceptualized as an incomplete elaboration of a phrase structure tree, with a premature appearance of representations at the noun and verb phrase level. If so, the nouns and verbs of agrammatic patients should not have precisely the same value as those same lexical units in normal speech. Certainly, agrammatics use nouns in a more diffuse, more propositional (holophrastic) way. Their difficulty in classifying nouns (Lhermitte et al., 1971) may reflect an attenuation of noun phrase differentiation. However, this is only a way of characterizing agrammatic language and may not reflect real psychological events. The preferential sparing of nouns and simple verbs in agrammatism may well have more to do with the initial use of these items as activity concepts, in relation to the cognitive mode of their acquisition. This is not to suggest that the agrammatic has a child's grammar; there is considerable evidence against this point of view. The evidence suggests, rather, that the young child's use of language in relation to activity may play a determining role in the psychological representation of these lexical items.

(Brown, 1979, pp. 179–181)

This rather long excerpt reinforces a developing bias of this author that seems shared with Vygotsky, Luria, and the line of Russian thinking that apparently originated with Bechterew and Pavlov (see discussion in Meader and Muyskens, 1950, pp. 207–209). The thesis is that the ontogeny of the speech-motor act (i.e., the child's emerging expressions of thought through speech) is a prime determinant of cognitive development (including semantics and pragmatics), leaving "language," per se, with only the syntactic content, i.e., the agreed upon rules of order for the emergence and differentiation of thought (see also Robinson, 1975). Surely the details of Brown's predictions will be revised as the appropriate clinical and neurobiologic data become available. Nonetheless, Brown's concept of the evolving "motor envelope" represents to me a beginning set of biologic-behavioral hypotheses about these processes—with a clear pointer to phylo-ontogenetic determinants of speech and thought as well as the neurosymptomatology that will appear according to the age of the patient and the locus of the lesion. Brown's additional points are that the lesion usually must be bilateral to be of clinical significance and that subcortical lesions are more devastating than cortical lesions.

Distributed Functions and Restricted Lesions

The studies of Darley and colleagues (1969a, 1969b) provided a springboard for physiology studies in the 1970s. Five perceptually distinct forms of dysarthria were identified, and hypotheses were formed regarding their pathologic neuroanatomy and neurophysiology. Netsell (Chapter 2) reviewed the physiology studies of the 1970s concerning flaccid, ataxic, and parkinsonian dysarthria. In this section, particular emphasis is given to the effects of lesions at various levels of the brainstem on speech function. These lesions and associated speech disturbances give further clues about the organization of speech neural mechanisms and point to the need for refinement as well as elaboration of current classifications of the dysarthrias.

For this discussion, the brainstem is defined as the medulla oblongata, pons, and midbrain (Warwick and Williams, 1973). In general, lesions restricted to the cranial nerves and cell bodies yield the classic signs of flaccid dysarthria (Darley et al., 1969a, 1969b), but even this "neurologic truism" may have exceptions. Bratzlavsky and vander Eecken (1977) believed their seven patients had undergone altered synaptic organization of the facial nucleus following facial nerve regeneration during recovery from Bell's palsy. The earlier flaccid signs were replaced by a "hemifacial hypertonia." So-called irritative brainstem lesions that act on the inputs of the cranial nerve nuclei also can yield symptoms of hypertonicity (Jankovic and Patel, 1983).

Congenital or acquired lesions in the lower brainstem (medulla and pons) that involve the reticular core result in hypertonic postures and reactions in the head, neck, torso, and limbs (Mysak, 1976, 1980). Netsell and Daniel (1979) speculated that their client showed "flaccid" signs in the orofacial system and "spastic" limbs as trauma residuals affecting the lower and upper motoneurons of the lower brainstem for the cranial and spinal motor systems, respectively.

Studies of the "locked in syndrome" (LiS) point to other restricted motor pathways of the rostral midbrain—for example, the rostral pons and cerebral peduncles at the lower midbrain (see reviews in Bauer, Gerstenbrand, and Rumpl, 1979; Bauer, Gerstenbrand, and Hengl, 1980). In its pure form, LiS permits no movement other than vertical deflections of the eyes. LiS patients signal with their eyes that they have sensory as well as considerable cognitive function, including one patient in whom the above-average cognition has been preserved for 12 years (Cappa and Vignolo, 1982). More typically, the LiS is incomplete and the patients vocalize to emotional stimuli and show limited movements of the limbs (Bauer et al., 1979, 1980).

These varieties of LiS suggest that limbic and perhaps reticular pathways also are involved. Although rare, recovery from LiS does occur (McCusker, Rudick, Honch, and Griggs, 1982). McCusker and colleagues documented four such cases and the early return of function was not predictive of a better overall recovery. All four patients were believed to have ventral pontine infarcts. Two of these subjects demonstrated trismus (tonic spasms of the jaw muscles). If the other two patients had subclinical trismus, it could be hypothesized that trismus resulted from upper motoneuron lesions of the trigeminal system as well as cranial nuclei below the pons. This could account for flaccid facial muscles and hypertonic, or "spastic," muscles whose cranial nuclei were inferior to the lesion. Alternatively, only muscles with spindles might show spasticity (see discussion in Barlow and Abbs, 1984).

Bauer, Prugger, and Rumpl (1982) report three cases of LiS demonstrating stimulus-evoked "oral automatisms." Although sucking and chewing movements never occurred spontaneously, these could be evoked with oral or perioral stimulation. The authors speculate that complete systems for sucking and chewing exist in the brainstem that can be evoked in the absence of cortical input.

Bilateral lesions involving corticobulbar and corticospinal pathways in the midbrain may yield the purer forms of pseudobulbar palsy. Lesions at this level may produce weakness and spasticity due to the direct and indirect cortical projections, respectively (Darley et al., 1975), and the pathologic crying and laughter due to limbic system damage. Higher lesions involving the thalamus and cortex are complicated by aphasia, apraxia, or both (Brown, 1979). Indeed, as suggested by Brodal (1973), unilateral involvement at the internal capsule may yield not only a dysarthria but a dyspraxia as well. More discussion of Brodal's case is found later in this chapter (see *Treating the Dysarthrias*).

The natural course of recovery following traumatic midbrain lesions offers further clues regarding the motor organization of speech. Vogel and von Cramon (1982) described voice recovery in eight patients with head trauma and sequelae that were hypothesized to result from compression of midbrain structures caused by cerebral swelling. An initial stage of mutism was accompanied by "affective" vocalizations (groaning, sighing, laughing, and crying) and involuntary coughs. The patients could produce no vocalization or other movement at will.

Of the six patients who were tested with the short form of the Token Test, an aphasic disorder could be excluded. The mutism was followed by a "whispery stage," lasting 1 to 3 weeks, in which "phonologically relevant movements appeared that were impaired in the majority of patients" (p. 153). In some patients, expiratory and inspiratory breathing patterns alternated from one syllable to the next, and "coughing, throat clearing, etc., could not be produced at will during this stage" (p. 153). There was a 2 to 3 week transition stage from whispered to "constant voiced production," in which voice production was variable, breathy, and reduced in loudness. Once a constant voice was achieved, all types of vocalization could be produced at will. "An appropriate loudness level during conversational speech was the first vocal parameter to reach normal limits" (p. 154). The remaining voice problems included a "limited ability to regulate pitch and the reduced pitch range," and the development of a "tense voice." The latter resembled spastic dysphonia and was believed to reflect a compensatory overcontraction of larnygeal adductor muscles. Commenting on some of the same patients, von Cramon (1981) noted

> During the transition between mutistic stage and the reappearance of verbal utterances patients produced central vowels and slides only, the first being "ja" (yes). Opening but also rounding and spreading of the lips were markedly restricted. As soon as consonants could be differentiated, patients showed a tendency to shift places of articulation posteriorly. An analysis of the manner of articulation revealed that the patients were not able to produce, and later to maintain, occlusions or stable constrictions. . . . The most salient feature, however, was the impaired motor control of the tongue tip. . . . The motor disturbance of the front part of the tongue persisted as long as the patients were observed. (p. 803)

Considering our earlier discussion of the lesion studies of squirrel monkeys, the vocalization recovery of these midbrain patients shows several parallels. As emotional vocalizations were possible in the mutistic stage, von Cramon (1981) assumed the periaqueductal gray matter had been spared. The general course of voice and speech recovery also recapitulated the normal acquisition of speech motor skill in normal infants and children, giving some credence to von Cramon's hypothesis that "the most likely explanation is that traumatic mutism is caused by a temporal inhibition of neural activity within the brainstem vocalization system."

Shared Versus Specialized Neuronal Mechanisms

Meader and Muyskens (1959) believed that speech motor functions were phylogenetic and ontogenetic differentiations of the more primitive functions of sucking, chewing, and swallowing. "Thus, we see that specific vegetative structures and functions arose through a process of fragmentation of the simpler peristaltic structures and functions. These newer functions formed the matrix from which the speech movements emerged" (p. 243).

Vocal tract movements for vowel and consonants were said to have emerged from fragmentation of the peristaltic wave (Meader and Muyskens, 1950; Shohara, 1932). The supporting data were drawn from x-ray similarities of tongue shapes during vowel productions and segments of the swallowing act (Shohara, 1932). Speech was said to be an "overlaid function" on these vegetative functions. Treatments evolved from this view, including a hierarchical scheme that sucking, swallowing, and chewing were determinants of and prerequisites for speech (e.g., see Crickmay, 1977; Fawcus, 1969). Among the clinical observations that reinforce the "overlaid" hypothesis are (1) speech is almost always severely involved when swallowing is a problem; (2) speech improves with improvement in swallowing; (3) chewing and swallowing can be normal and speech severely dysarthric; and (4) the act of simultaneous chewing and speaking is reported to improve speech when attempts to speak without chewing are unsuccessful.

All of the necessary neuronal machinery for these vegetative acts is located within the brainstem. Cortical motoneurons may participate in certain aspects of chewing, but they are not necessary. The hypothesis is that sucking and swallowing are phylogenetically older and controlled by reticulolimbic structures of the brainstem. Chewing has evolved more recently and, with the appearance of teeth, may require sensorimotor interactions of the tongue and jaw that are antecedents to tongue-jaw neuronal mechanisms used in speaking. Our ancestors undoubtedly vocalized while chewing and heard more differentiated sound patterns from the tongue movements. These "new sounds" may have become a way to signal more discrete units of "meaning" in their communication and may have been the origins of tongue movements for speech. Studies of tooth eruption and the differentiation of tongue movements for speech in individual infants may show a similar progression.

The point of the foregoing is to suggest that the neuronal mechanisms for speech are not simply "overlaid" on those of vegetation any more than the neocortical system is overlaid on the limbic or reticular systems. All oromotor functions are impaired when shared or adjacent neuronal structures (e.g., cranial nerves or cranial nuclei) are damaged. Damage to brainstem pathways can interrupt fibers of all afferent-efferent systems. The alternative to the overlaid hypothesis is, that with the emergence of the neocortical system, the human sends unique commands to the lower motoneurons for speech and other fine motor skills. These may or may not be the same cell bodies and axons activated during vegetative acts. Regardless, both the patterns of activation and loci of the "command neurons" are specialized and differential for the motor acts of speech versus sucking, chewing, and swallowing.

Recovery from Brain Injury

Recent reviews reveal that many brain injured patients can show remarkable improvements beyond the usual 2 years, and various forms of treatment (including behavioral therapies) can facilitate the natural recovery processes (Bach-y-Rita, 1980; Finger and Stein, 1982). Wall's summary (1980) draws attention to the many factors involved in recovery and suggests factors that can and cannot be assumed to be of influence.

> We began with the fact that those who survive brain damage show a surprising degree of recovery. No doubt some of this recovery is to be attributed to readjustments of blood vessels and other factors on which the brain depends. However, some degree of recovery is seen even where there is known permanent destruction of parts of the central nervous system. Certain mechanisms cannot be proposed to explain the recovery. Brain cells in the adult do not divide to reproduce new cells. Nerve fibres cut across in the central nervous system do not regenerate as they do in the periphery. Certain suggestions to explain recovery are rejected as being unhelpful and mystical since they do not specify what it is that has changed during recovery. Words such as shock, diaschisis and redundancy are not useful. There is no doubt that the patient learns to substitute alternative mechanisms for those he has lost just as a blind man develops his skills of hearing and feeling and just as an amputee extends the repertoire of his remaining limbs. Beyond this crucial learning there are signs of unlearned readjustments within the brain. Nerve cells show a type of homeostasis so that if they lose part of their input, they adjust their excitability to capture fully the excitatory effects of their remaining input. Where nerve fibres degenerate, the nearby intact fibres have an ability to sprout and occupy the site left vacant by the degenerated fibres. Beyond this sprouting mechanism there are large numbers of normally ineffective nerve connections which may become active if the dominant inputs are out of action. It is proposed that the connections laid down in the embryo are more diffuse than those actually used in the adult brain. The stage of maturation involves partly destruction of the "incorrect" connections and partly their suppression. If some nervous connections are destroyed in the adult, suppressed connections may become depressed. This process is not necessarily a good thing; the substituted connections may bring in nonsense information which the recovering nervous system cannot handle. Sprouting and the unmasking of ineffective connections offers the possibility of new connections after brain damage, but we need to know much more about these processes so that we can guide them to useful ends rather than toward further disorganisation. (pp. 103–104)

TREATING THE DYSARTHRIAS

Incorporating much of the foregoing discussion, suggestions and hypotheses are offered for consideration in treating the individual with dysarthria. It will be obvious that these are matters for research, rather than data-based clinical procedures or recommendations.

Factors Influencing Treatment Outcome

In considering treatment for the individual with dysarthria, several factors influence the eventual level of speech production skill that can be expected. These factors include (1) neurologic status and history, (2) age, (3) "automatic" adjustments, (4) treatment effects, (5) personality and intelligence, and (6) support systems.

Neurologic Status and History

The overriding factor influencing motor performance in general, and speech production in particular, would seem to be the location, extent, and underlying neuropathology of the lesion or lesions. As reviewed earlier in this chapter, bilateral subcortical or brainstem lesions seem most devastating and least reversible. Less massive lesions to cortical aspects of the neocortical system offer a better prognosis, and even unilateral left brain lesions sparing subcortical structures have optimistic outcomes. The issue of neuropathology is most critical in cases of degenerative disease (e.g., amyotrophic lateral sclerosis or dystonia musculorum deformans). Even in these cases, however, the deterioration can be gradual over a number of years and both biomedical and behavioral treatments can help in maintaining communication skills. The human nervous system has remarkable capabilities to work around or through lesions. Even though lesions place certain limits on performance, only the most severe (e.g., those causing an unremitting mutism) would appear to be unresponsive to therapeutic intervention.

The individual's neurologic history also is an obvious consideration. The adult with a developmental dysarthria (e.g., cerebral palsy) has different needs in terms of speech motor learning than one who was neurologically normal before insult. A young school-age child with head injury who was progressing normally would seem to need a different treatment program from a youngster with a history of developmental disability. Even though knowledge of the premorbid history is critical, it is often overlooked or unavailable.

Age

Given the course of neural maturation just outlined, persons experiencing neurologic insults following early but incomplete development of the neocortical system (say, perhaps, after age 2 or 3) might be expected to have, or to develop, better speech motor skills than those whose lesions occurred earlier. Lenneberg (1968) reports that many infants with cortical and lesser subcortical lesions appear symptom-free until the first or second year, when they "grow into" the lesion. The implication is that intact reticulolimbic systems can support the more innate early motor skills. Problems with learned motor skills become evident as the neocortical system fails to develop. Younger children have a better chance to "grow out of" or "around" their lesions than adults, presumably because the children's developing neuronal connectivities are more plastic. Elderly patients, on the other hand, would seem most negatively affected by the age variable since their nervous systems are deteriorating as a natural process. However, a recent case study of an 83 year old patient who used EMG feedback to relieve chronic facial spasm illustrates that even the severely involved geriatric patient can benefit from carefully planned treatment (Rubow, Rosenbek, Collins, and Celesia, 1984).

Automatic Adjustments

In response to a lesion, the individual makes a variety of automatic adjustments; some are adaptive and others are maladaptive. Some are intended and others are unintended, reactive, or "obligatory" as a consequence of the neuropathology. A major task for the clinician is to identify these automatic adjustments during the evaluation period, incorporating those that are useful in developing or restoring speech and removing or minimizing those that are not.

Treatment Effects

Obviously the selection of treatments (whether medical, physical, behavioral, or some combination) can affect speech production. Unfortunately, the selection of treatments usually reflects the educational and experience biases of the clinician as opposed to what is objectively the most efficacious treatment. Fortunately, the adaptive and robust nature of the nervous system allows most clients to improve their speech, regardless of clinician bias. In the absence of data on comparative treatments, it is this writer's opinion that almost any speech therapy for a dysarthric client is helpful; few *speech* therapies are directly harmful; and the "whatever works" approach will continue to dominate most therapies until we learn more about the physiology and neuropathophysiology of speech. Basic and clinical researchers must join in these studies of the speech mechanism and the differential response of the dysarthric client to various treatments.

A related problem is that often the combined efforts of the physician, speech clinician, and occupational and physical therapists are not optimally coordinated. Even when speech appears not to be a primary concern, the speech clinician must know the helpful or deleterious effects on speech of the treatments provided by the other disciplines. For example, bilateral ventrolateral thalamic surgery can relieve tremor, rigidity, or dystonia in the limbs and leave the patient with a persistent, often severe, dysarthria (Cooper, 1969).

Personality and Intelligence

A major influence on the eventual intelligibility of speech for the dysarthric client is his or her premorbid personality and intelligence. In my experience, the most dominant factor is personality, and those who were optimistic and purposeful before injury have a clear advantage over those who were not. Establishing the premorbid intelligence is important in considering treatment objectives and outcomes when there is cause to suspect subnormal levels prior to injury.

Support Systems

The ongoing treatment and carry-over of skills are enhanced for the brain-injured patient when there are "significant others" in his or her life and the prospects for making contributions to society, however modest, are realistic. Again, in my experience, these individuals have a much better prognosis for maintaining intelligible speech or optimizing use of augmentative communication aids. For a review of augmentative communication systems, see Linebaugh, Baird, Baird, and Armour (1983).

The Effects of Treatment for the Dysarthrias

Earlier beliefs that most unintelligible dysarthric patients were restricted to this condition for life have been dispelled for the most part by a number of case studies. Whereas recent advances in neurochemical treatments are more obvious (e.g., see Coyle, 1983), those in clinical speech treatments seem less well recognized by other disciplines. Most new colleagues I meet in medicine (e.g., neurology, pediatrics, rehabilitation medicine, and otolaryngology) or neuroscience are unaware that even severely impaired dysarthric subjects can respond to behavioral interventions. Indeed, even many speech clinicians are unaware of behavioral interventions or are unprepared to be helpful with severe cases.

A Neurophysiologic Emphasis

Although the obvious goal is to improve speech intelligibility, acceptability, or both, the most efficacious demonstrations of change are accompanied by physiologic or neurophysiologic recordings. These recordings are imperative in attempting to normalize a subsystem (e.g., respiratory) when no immediate increase in intelligibility is to be expected (e.g., see Abbs, Hunker, and Barlow, 1983; Netsell and Daniel, 1979; Rosenbek and LaPointe, 1978). Perhaps the most powerful paradigm for the immediate future will be case studies that incorporate clinical (neurologic and speech), neurochemical, and physiologic or neurophysiologic data. For an example of this in the neurology literature, see Chadwick, Hallett, and Harris (1977). Concerning the clinical speech data, it is imperative to document changes in speech intelligibility or acceptability.

Perceptual and Acoustic Documentation of Speech Changes

Perceptual ratings of speech intelligibility are most valid when evaluated by listeners unfamiliar with the speaker or subject matter (context) of the spoken material. This is easily achieved by having uninvolved staff members rate edited samples of the client's conversation. Documenting the contributing changes in articulation skill, speaking rate, and so on, can be done by the speech specialists (e.g., using the rating scales of Darley et al., 1975) or measurements of speech acoustics (e.g., see Weismer, 1984; Weismer and Cariski, 1984), or both.

Choice of Treatments

The treatments that have persisted over the years have been based upon particular neurophysiologic hypotheses (e.g., neurodevelopmental treatment, neuromuscular facilitation, the motokinesthetic method). Treatment procedures and their sequencing are developed from these hypotheses, but very little (if any) behavioral or physiologic data are available to demonstrate the effectiveness of a given procedure, or its advantage over an alternative procedure. In the absence of these data, it is difficult to recommend a given treatment at the expense of another. Many clinicians are forced to develop an eclectic approach that incorporates features of different theories or methods. Recent advances in physiologic recordings during speech should be helpful in remedying this situation.

Lessons from Brodal

Brodal's (1973) reflections on his recovery following a stroke suggest that almost all the treatments offered him were of some value. He also was impressed that a right hemisphere lesion had disturbing effects on motor control of the same (ipsilateral) body side. No clinical evidence of aphasia was found, but he described problems with short-term memory and apraxic-like errors in writing and speaking. During speech, "sometimes a word was skipped or a syllable, especially at the end of a sentence, or two small words were incorrectly fused" (p. 686). He hypothesized that the dysarthria, which persisted for at least 10 months, resulted from the asymmetry of bilateral innervation, and destruction of ipsilateral corticofugal fibers, including corticopontine fibers, which he estimated to outnumber pyramidal fibers by approximately 19 to 1. Brodal also speculated the dysarthria was related to a disturbance of cerebellar influence, via pontocere-bellothalamic connections. As Brodal points out, only autopsy will verify that no left hemisphere lesion existed and that his lesion was restricted to the right internal capsule. Regardless, his thoughts about lost and recovered functions following stroke are among the most informative ever written. Even though the paragraphs that follow relate to Brodal's problems in regaining use of the extremities, the parallels in restoring the motor control for speech appear to be strong.

The Value of Passive Movements. In addition to helping maintain a full range of motion in the joints, Brodal thought the passive movements of the physical therapist helped him initiate and direct the desired movement.

> Subjectively, it was clearly felt as if the sensory information produced by the passive movement helped the patient to "direct" the "force of innervation" through the proper channels. . . . It may well be that there are subtle neuro-physiological mechanisms involved in this "facilitation" of movements. From introspection it appears, however, that the subjective information about the movement to be executed, its range and goal, is an essential factor. The phenomenon is probably parallel to the learning of all motor skills. Among an original multitude of more or less haphazard movements, the correct ones are recognized as such by means of the sensory information they feed back to the central nervous system, and this information is later used in selecting the correct movements in the further training. (p. 678)

Skilled Movements. Brodal illustrated his loss of skilled movement by describing problems in tying his bow tie, a skill he had used daily for some 40 years.

> The appropriate finger movements were difficult to perform with sufficient strength, speed and coordination, but it was quite obvious to the patient that the main reason for failure was something else.
> Under normal conditions the necessary numerous small delicate movements had followed each other in proper sequence almost automatically, and the act of tying when first started had proceeded without much conscious attention. Subjectively, the patient felt as if he had to stop because "his fingers did not know the next move." He had the same feeling as when one recites a poem or sings a song and gets lost. The only way is to start from the beginning. It was felt as if the delay in the succession of movements (due to paresis and spasticity) interrupted a chain of more or less automatic move-

ments. Consciously directing attention to the finger movements did not improve the performance, on the contrary it made it quite impossible (p. 679)

Force of Innervation. A final problem of Brodal's that may relate to speech rehabilitation was with what he termed the "force of innervation."

> It was a striking and repeatedly made observation that the force needed to make a severely paretic muscle contract is considerable. The expression of this force in this connection refers to what one, for the lack of a better expression, might call force of innervation. Subjectively, this is experienced as a kind of mental force, a power of will. In the case of a muscle just capable of being actively moved, the mental effort needed was very great. The greater the degree of paresis of such a muscle, the greater was the mental effort needed to make it contract and to oppose voluntarily even a very weak counter-force. On the other hand, only a slight mental effort was needed to bring about a fairly good contraction of a muscle able to work with about half or a little less of its full force. (p. 677)

Speech Therapy. Brodal did not mention receiving any formal speech therapy. It may be that his speech recovery, which took at least 10 months, was essentially due to natural recovery. It may be that his recovery would have been accelerated by certain behavioral procedures. For example, the use of lip force or EMG feedback might have been helpful in the early stages of weakness, where movement could not be "willed." This might have allowed him to reestablish afferent-to-efferent relationships earlier, as well as initiate muscle contractions more rapidly. Brodal believed the loss of sequencing skilled movements was not due simply to problems with strength, speed, and coordination; rather, he pointed to the loss of automaticity in sequencing. Given earlier discussion in this chapter about the importance of instantaneous afference in the regulation, if not construction, of individual spatial-temporal goals, it is hypothesized that "getting lost" in a sequence is caused by a reduction in speed of movement associated with individual goal achievement. That is, the quantity and quality of afference generated during the slow movements may be confusing or insufficient for achievement of the intended goal and the speaker does not move on automatically to the next goal.

In other cases of severe dysarthria, the force or EMG feedback work could be tried (1) when no speech was possible, (2) as an adjunct to speech initiation, or (3) when attempting movements for individual spatial-temporal goals.

Shared and Specialized Mechanisms

The extent to which the neural mechanisms of speech share the phylogenetic or ontogenetic mechanisms used for sucking, chewing, or swallowing is a matter for further research. Feeding therapy undoubtedly helps some children to feed better, and may even facilitate vocalization development (Morris, 1980). The inhibition of detrimental postural reactions, careful presentation of graded orofacial stimuli, and other means to counteract "primitive behavior" may all facilitate speech development. But, it does not necessarily follow that these are antecedents to, or prerequisites for, the neural connectivities developed for or used in speaking. In the absence of data, perhaps a conservative blend of theory and practice is most appropriate in the clinic. For example, consider treating a presumed antecedent behavior when the more recently evolved or acquired behavior is not present. When the antecedents are believed to be necessary prerequisites, consider treating the highest level available of the desired skill (speech) simultaneously with the available level of the antecedent behavior. For example, "chewing therapy" may facilitate speech not because it's a phylogenetic or ontogenetic determinant, but because (1) it generates afferent consequences of oromotor movements (when speech cannot), (2) it forces speech motor equivalence during the chewing act, or (3) the afference generated during chewing engages neuronal connections that are common to both chewing and speech.

Consider the thesis that speech and other fine motor skills are a "quantum leap" beyond earlier structure and function. This quantum leap is not a discontinuity in evolution, but an acceleration that yields clear advantages in adapting to the present environment and shaping its future. Clinically, this line of thinking might translate to the following question: Would you ask Philippe Entremont (classical pianist), in attempting to regain the motor skill of piano playing, to begin at any skill level *below* the most advanced he could demonstrate during testing?

Carry-Over from Clinic to the Outside

The transfer of the speaking skills obtained in the clinic to "real world" situations is a much needed area of research. The incorporation of "real world" speaking skills, situations, and strategies for maintaining them need to be introduced in clinic work at the earliest appropriate time.

EPILOGUE

In many (if not most) respects, Luria encompassed 25 years ago the ideas presented in this neurobiologic view of the dysarthrias. It is of interest that toward the end of his life he was planning to study the subcortical influences of speech, language, and thought, with special emphasis on neurochemical mechanisms.

The basic theme of this chapter has been that nothing is *static*—not the organism itself, its behavior, or its response to lesion or treatment. A neurobiologic view is at once converging and diverging. The *convergence* is seen in the neurologic reductionism to understand the organism's behavior in terms of its present (and past) structure and function. The *divergence* is in the brain and behavior of the organism, where continued differentiation of thought and elaboration of the nervous system remind us of our potential for growth. Little has been said of so-called psychologic functions because they are believed to be biologic ones not yet understood.

ACKNOWLEDGMENTS

Preparation of this manuscript was supported by the Boys Town National Institute and an NIH research grant (NS 16763). L. D'Antonio and J. Rosenbek made helpful editorial comments and C. Dugan provided her usual excellence in manuscript preparation.

REFERENCES

Abbs, J., and Cole, K. (1982). Consideration of bulbar and suprabulbar afferent influences upon speech motor coordination and programming. In S. Grillner, B. Lindblom, J. Lubker and A. Persson (Eds.), *Speech motor control*. New York: Pergamon Press.

Abbs, J. H., and Gracco, V.L. (1984). Sensorimotor actions in the control of multimovement speech gestures. *Trends in Neuroscience, 6*(9), 391–395.

Abbs, J., Hunker, C. J., and Barlow, S. M. (1983). Differential speech motor subsystem impairments with suprabulbar lesions: Neurophysiological framework and supporting data. In W. Berry (Ed.), *Clinical dysarthria*. San Diego: College-Hill Press.

Abbs, J. H., and Kennedy, J. (1980). Neurophysiological processes of speech movement control. In N. Lass, J. Northern, D. Yoder, and L. McReynolds (Eds.), *Speech, language, and hearing*. Philadelphia: W. B. Saunders.

Bach-y-Rita, P. (1980). *Recovery of function: Theoretical considerations for brain injury rehabilitation*. Baltimore: University Park Press.

Barlow, S. M., and Abbs, J. H. (1984). Orofacial fine motor control impairments in congenital spasticity: Evidence against hypertonus related performance deficits. *Journal of Neurology, 34*, 145–150.

Bauer, G., Gerstenbrand, F., and Hengl, W. (1980). Involuntary motor phenomena in the locked-in syndrome. *Journal of Neurology, 223*, 191–198.

Bauer, G., Gerstenbrand, F., and Rumpl, E. (1979). Varieties of the locked-in syndrome. *Journal of Neurology, 221*, 77–91.

Bauer, G., Prugger, M., and Rumpl, E. (1982). Stimulus evoked oral automatisms in the locked-in syndrome. *Archives of Neurology, 39*, 435–436.

Bauer, H., Kent, R., and Murray, A. (1983). *Ethologic perspectives on first word development*. Paper presented to the Midwest Regional Animal Behavior Meeting, St. Louis.

Bratzlavsky, M., and vander Eecken, H. (1977). Altered synaptic organization in facial nucleus following facial nerve regeneration: An electrophysiological study in man. *Annals of Neurology, 2,* 71–73.

Brodal, A. (1973). Self-observations and neuro-anatomical considerations after a stroke. *Brain, 96,* 675–694.

Brown, J. (1975). On the neural organization of language: Thalamic and cortical relationships. *Brain and Language, 2,* 18–30.

Brown, J. (1979). Language representation in the brain. In H. Steklis and M. Raleigh (Eds.), *Neurobiology of social communication in primates: An evolutionary perspective.* New York: Academic Press.

Canter, G. J. (1963). Speech characteristics of patients with Parkinson's disease: I. Intensity, pitch and duration. *Journal of Speech and Hearing Disorders, 28,* 221–229.

Canter, G. J. (1965a). Speech characteristics of patients with Parkinson's disease: II. Physiological support for speech. *Journal of Speech and Hearing Disorders, 30,* 44–49.

Canter, G. J. (1965b). Speech characteristics of patients with Parkinson's disease: III. Articulation, diadochokinesis, and overall speech adequacy. *Journal of Speech and Hearing Disorders, 30,* 217–224.

Cappa, S., and Vignolo, L. (1982). Locked-in syndrome for 12 years with preserved intelligence. *Annals of Neurology, 11,* 545.

Chadwick, D., Hallett, M., and Harris, R. (1977). Clinical, biochemical and physiological factors distinguishing myoclonus responsive to 5-hydroxy-tryptophan, tryptophan plus a monoamine oxidase inhibitor and clonazepam. *Brain, 100,* 455–487.

Cole, K. (1981). *An empirical re-evaluation of minimum voluntary afferent-to-efferent pathway latencies in the orofacial system.* Unpublished master's thesis, University of Wisconsin, Madison.

Cooper, I. (1969). *Involuntary movement disorders.* New York: Harper & Row.

Coyle, J. (1983). *Neurotransmitter systems in psychotic and cognitive behavior.* Paper presented to the Symposium on Developmental Disabilities V: Autism and Related Disorders of Communication. Johns Hopkins Medical Center, Baltimore.

Cramon, D. von (1981). Traumatic mutism and the subsequent reorganization of speech functions. *Neurophyschologia, 19,* 801–805.

Crickmay, M. (1977). *Speech therapy and the bobath approach to cerebral palsy.* Springfield, IL: Charles C Thomas.

Darley, F. L., Aronson, A. E., and Brown, J. R. (1969a). Differential diagnostic patterns of dysarthria. *Journal of Speech and Hearing Research, 12,* 246–269.

Darley, F. L., Aronson, A. E., and Brown, J. R. (1969b). Clusters of deviant speech dimensions in the dysarthrias. *Journal of Speech and Hearing Research, 12,* 462–496.

Darley, F. L., Aronson, A. E., and Brown, J. R. (1975). *Motor speech disorders.* Philadelphia: W.B. Saunders.

Evarts, E. (1982). Analogies between central motor programs for speech and for limb movements. In S. Grillner, B. Lindblom, J. Lubker, and A. Persson (Eds.), *Speech motor control.* New York: Pergamon Press.

Fawcus, B. (1969). Oropharyngeal function in relation to speech. *Developmental Medicine and Child Neurology, 11,* 556–560.

Ferrendelli, J. (1983). Neuropharmacology. Short course presented to the 35th meeting of the American Academy of Neurology, San Diego.

Finger, S., and Stein, D. (1982). *Brain damage and recovery: Research and clinical perspectives.* New York: Academic Press.

Fromm, D. (1981). *Investigation of movement/EMG parameters in apraxia of speech.* Unpublished master's thesis, University of Wisconsin, Madison.

Goldstein, K. (1915). *Die transkortikalen Aphasien.* Jene: Fischer.

Grillner, S. (1982). Possible analogies in the contol of innate motor acts and the production of speech. In S. Grillner, B. Lindblom, J. Lubker, and A. Persson (Eds.), *Speech motor control.* New York: Pergamon Press.

Hammarberg, R. (1982). On redefining coarticulation. *Journal of Phonetics, 10,* 123–137.

Hardy, J. (1964). Lung function of atheroid and spastic quadriplegic children. *Developmental Medicine and Child Neurology, 6,* 378–388.

Hardy, J. (1966). Suggestions for physiological research in dysarthria. *Cortex, 3,* 128–156.

Hardy, J. (1970). Development of neuromuscular systems underlying speech production. In *Speech and the dentofacial complex: The state of the art. ASHA Reports,* No. 5, 49–68.

Harris, F. (1969). Control of gamma efferents through the reticular activating system. *American Journal of Occupational Therapy, 23,* 397–409.

Harris, F. (1971). Inapproprioception: A possible sensory basis for athetoid movements. *Journal of the American Physical Therapy Association, 51.*

Hunker, C. J., and Abbs, J. H. (1984). Physiological analyses of parkinsonian tremors in the orofacial system. In M. R. McNeil, J. C. Rosenbek, and A. E. Aronson (Eds.), *The dysarthrias: Physiology, acoustics, perception, and management.* San Diego: College-Hill Press.

Hunker, C., Abbs, J., and Barlow, S. (1982). The relationship between parkinsonian rigidity and hypokinesia in the orofacial system: A quantitative analysis. *Neurology, 32,* 755–761.

Jankovic, J., and Patel, C. (1983). Brainstem origin of blepharospasm. *Neurology, 33* (Suppl 2), 162.

Johnston, M., and Coyle, J. (1981). Development of central neurotransmitter systems. In *The fetus and independent life* (Ciba Foundation Symposium 86), London: Pitman.

Jurgens, U. (1979). Neural control of vocalization in nonhuman primates. In H. Steklis and M. Raleigh (Eds.), *Neurobiology of social communication in primates.* New York: Academic Press.

Kent, R. (1973). Cinefluorographic studies of dysarthria (Research Grant NS-11022). Bethesda, MD: National Institutes of Health.

Kent, R. (1981). Articulatory-acoustic perspectives on speech development. In R. Stark (Ed.), *Language behavior in infancy and early childhood.* New York: Elsevier/North-Holland.

Kent, R. (1984). Brain mechanisms of speech and language with special reference to emotional interactions. In R. Naremore (Ed.), *Language science.* San Diego: College-Hill Press.

Lenneberg, E. (1967). *Biological foundations of language.* New York: Wiley & Sons.

Lenneberg, E. (1968). The effect of age on the outcome of central nervous system disease in children. In R. Isaacson (Ed.), *The neuropsychology of development.* New York: Wiley & Sons.

Lhermitte, F., Derouesne, J., and Lecours, A. (1971). Contribution to the study of semantic disorders in aphasia. *Revue Neurologique, 125,* 81–101.

Linebaugh, C., Baird, J., Baird, C., and Armour, R. (1983). Special considerations for the development of microcomputer-based augmentative communication systems. In W. Berry (Ed.), *Clinical dysarthria.* San Diego: College-Hill Press.

Logemann, J., Fisher, H., Boshes, B., and Blonsky, E. (1978). Frequency and co-occurrence of vocal tract dysfunction in the speech of a large sample of Parkinson patients. *Journal of Speech and Hearing Disorders, 43,* 47–57.

Lubker, J. (1982). Spatio-temporal goals: Maturational and cross-linguistic variables. In S. Grillner, B. Lindblom, J. Lubker, and A. Persson (Eds.), *Speech motor control.* New York: Pergamon Press.

Luria, A. (1970). *Traumatic aphasia.* The Hague, Netherlands: Mouton.

Luria, A. (1981). *Language and cognition.* New York: Wiley & Sons.

MacLean, P. (1970). The triune brain, emotion and scientific bias. In F. Schmitt (Ed.), *The neurosciences: Second study program.* New York: Rockefeller University Press.

McCusker, E., Rudick, R., Honch, G., and Griggs, R. (1982). Recovery from the locked-in syndrome. *Archives of Neurology, 39,* 145–147.

Meader, C., and Muyskens, J. (1950). *Handbook of biolinguistics, part 1: The structures and processes of expression.* Baltimore: Waverly Press.

Moore, J. (1980). Neuroanatomical considerations relating to recovery of function following brain injury. In P. Bach-y-Rita (Ed.), *Recovery of function: Theoretical considerations for brain injury rehabilitation.* Baltimore: University Park Press.

Morris, S. (1980). *Pre-speech assessment scale: A rating scale for the measurement of pre-speech behaviors from birth through two years.* Milwaukee: Cerebral Palsy Project-Curative Rehabilitation Center.

Mountcastle, V. (1978). An organizing principle for cerebral function: The unit module and the distributed system. In G. Edleman and V. Mountcastle (Eds.), *The mindful brain.* Cambridge, MA: MIT Press.

Müller, E., Abbs, J., and Kennedy, J. (1981). Some systems physiology considerations for vocal control. In M. Hirano and K. Stevens (Eds.), *Vocal fold physiology.* Tokyo: University of Tokyo Press.

Muyskens, J. (1925). *The hypha.* Doctoral dissertation, University of Michigan, Ann Arbor.

Mysak, E. (1976). *Pathologies of speech systems.* Baltimore: Williams & Wilkins.

Mysak, E. (1980). *Neurospeech therapy for the cerebral palsied: A neuroevolutional approach.* New York: Teachers College Press.

Netsell, R. (1971). Physiological bases of dysarthria (Research Grant NS09627). Bethesda, MD: National Institutes of Health.

Netsell, R., and Daniel, B. (1979). Dysarthria in adults: Physiologic approach to rehabilitation. *Archives of Physical Medicine and Rehabilitation, 60,* 502–508.

Oller, D. (1981). Infant vocalizations: Exploration and reflexivity. In R. Stark (Ed.), *Language behavior in infancy and early childhood.* New York: Elsevier/North-Holland.

Penfield, W., and Roberts, L. (1959). *Speech and brain mechanisms.* Princeton, NJ: University Press.

Perkell, J., and Nelson, W. (1982). Articulatory targets and speech motor control: A study of vowel production. In S. Grillner, B. Lindblom, J. Lubker, and A. Persson (Eds.), *Speech motor control.* New York: Pergamon Press.

Peterson, G., and Shoup, J. (1966). A physiologic theory of phonetics. *Journal of Speech and Hearing Research, 9,* 5–67.

Ploog, D. (1979). Phonation, emotion, cognition, with reference to the brain mechanisms involved. *Ciba Foundation Symposium, 69,* 78–98.

Ploog, D. (1981). On the neural control of mammalian vocalization. *Trends in Neuroscience, 4,* 135–137.

Pribram, K. (1982). Brain mechanism in music: Prolegomena for a theory of meaning. In M. Clynes (Ed.), *Music, mind and brain: The neuropschology of music.* New York: Plenum Press, pp. 21–35.

Rieber, R. (1980). *Language development and aphasia in children.* New York: Academic Press.

Robinson, I. (1975). *The new grammarians' funeral: A critique of Noam Chomsky's linguistics.* New York: Cambridge University Press.

Rosenbek, J., and LaPointe, L. (1978). The dysarthrias: Description, diagnosis, and treatment. In D. F. Johns (Ed.), *Clinical management of communicative disorders.* Boston: Little, Brown.

Rosenberg, R. (1983). Clinical neurochemistry. Short course presented to the 35th Meeting of the American Academy of Neurology, San Diego.

Rubow, R. (1980). Biofeedback and the treatment of speech disorders. Biofeedback Society of America, Wheat Ridge, CO.

Rubow, R. T., Rosenbek, J. C., Collins, M. J., and Celesia, G. G. (1984). Reduction in hemifacial spasm and dysarthria following EMG feedback. *Journal of Speech and Hearing Disorders, 49,* 26–33.

Rutherford, D. (1967). Auditory-motor learning and the acquisition of speech. *American Journal of Physical Medicine, 46,* 245–251.

Shohara, H. (1932). *Genesis of articulatory movements in speech.* Doctoral dissertation, University of Michigan, Ann Arbor.

Shohara, H. (1939). Significance of overlapping movements in speech. *Proceedings of the Second Biennial Central Zone Conference of the American Society of the Hard of Hearing.*

Stetson, R. (1950). *Motor phonetics.* Amsterdam: North-Holland.

Tinbergen, N. (1963). On the aims and methods of ethology. *Zeit. t. Tierpsychol.,* 410–433.

Vogel, M., and Cramon, D. von (1982). Dysphonia after traumatic midbrain damage: A follow-up study. *Folia Phoniatrica, 34,* 150–159.

Wall, P. D. (1980). Mechanisms of plasticity of connection following damage in adult mammalian nervous systems. In P. Bach-y-Rita (Ed.), *Recovery of function: Theoretical considerations for brain injury rehabilitation.* Baltimore: University Park Press.

Warwick, R., and Williams, P. (1973). *Gray's anatomy.* Philadelphia: W. B. Saunders.

Weismer, G. (1984). Articulatory characteristics in parkinsonian dysarthria: Segmental and phrase-level timing, spirantization and glottal-supraglottal coordination. In M. R. MacNeil, J. C. Rosenbek, and A. E. Aronson, *The dysarthrias: Physiology, acoustics, perception, and management.* San Diego: College-Hill Press.

Weismer, G., and Cariski, D. (1984). On speakers' abilities to control speech mechanism output: Theoretical and clinical implications. In N. Lass (Ed.), *Speech and language: Advances in basic research and practice* (Vol. 10). New York: Academic Press.

Wolff, P. (1979). Theoretical issues in the development of motor skills. *Symposium on Developmental Disabilities in the Pre-School Child.* Chicago: Johnson & Johnson.

Wolff, P. (1981). Normal variation in human maturation. In K. Connolly and H. Prechtl (Eds.), *Maturation and development: Biological and psychological perspectives.* Philadelphia: J. B. Lippincott.

Yorkston, K. M., and Beukelman, D. R. (1981). Ataxic dysarthria: Treatment sequences based on intelligibility and prosodic considerations. *Journal of Speech and Hearing Disorders, 46,* 398–404.

Chapter **4**

Speech Motor Control: Theoretical Issues with Clinical Impact

In the past 10 to 15 years, expanded literatures have appeared on (1) the mechanisms of speech motor control in normal and neurologically impaired individuals, and (2) understanding and treating the dysarthrias (see Abbs and Cole, 1982; Hixon, 1982; Netsell, 1982, for reviews). Another literature dealing with the motor control of other body parts (e.g., the eyes, arms, hands, and legs) in humans and other mammals, is increasing even more rapidly (see Brooks, 1981). In the space available, I have rather presumptuously taken on the task of reviewing some of the current themes and issues of motor control that relate to the dysarthrias. for purposes of this presentation, *speech motor control* is broadly defined as the neuronal actions that initiate and regulate muscle contractions for speech production. The *speech motor system* refers to the neural mechanisms used to produce speech. From the host of topics that could be presented, I have selected ones that most directly influence how I think about speech as a motor skill and how that, in turn, affects my conceptualization of the motor control problem of the dysarthric client under study. Obviously, the questions we ask about what is going wrong with the speech of this person

Reprinted by permission of the publisher from *Clinical dysarthria,* W. Berry (Ed.), pp. 1–19. Copyright 1983 by College-Hill Press, Inc., San Diego, California.

are powerfully conditioned by (1) the way we believe normal speech is produced, (2) what goes wrong, from a motor control point of view, when given pathways or regions of the nervous system are damaged, and (3) when (in a developmental sense) the damage occurred. It seems likely that most dysarthric movement patterns combine the direct motor control effects of the lesion(s), secondary effects of altered postural reflexes (e.g., overall increases or decreases in muscle stiffness), and tertiary effects of intended, or unintended, compensatory adjustments. This raises the question of the extent to which models of normal speech production are applicable to the motor control problems facing the dysarthric speakers. This question, along with all others raised in this chapter, are basically unanswered. Even though the present answers are fuzzy, the asking of the questions serves several important purposes. First, we squarely face the facts versus fantasies of our current answers. Second, we try to restate the questions in terms of hypotheses for experimental tests. Third, we gauge the impact of these questions and answers on each part of our clinical practice.

METRICS OF NORMAL SPEECH

Precision Capabilities

We have the capability to reach highly precise successions of vocal tract shapes, seeming to reach acoustically critical points at critical points in time. That is, we often come within 1 mm of previously attained positions and time the phrasing of one articulator movement within 10 ms of another (Kent and Moll, 1975; Netsell, Kent, and Abbs, 1980). These spatial-temporal goals are reached rapidly, interactively (with respect to articulator trade-offs or "motor equivalence"), and are accomplished automatically (that is, without the conscious awareness of the speaker). This "motor equivalence" is accomplished in the upper airway through automatic velocity and directional changes in the articulator movements (see review in Abbs and Cole, 1982; Netsell et al., 1980). Additional trade-offs are made in the components of the respiratory system for maintaining a constant subglottal air pressure (Hixon, 1982). These adjustments in goal achievement are made in natural speech in response to small, externally applied loads, or in holding one part of the mechanism in a fixed position. Compared to our fastest movements (for example, those of the eyes), speech is relatively slow, probably using relatively small percentages of the muscles' maximum contractile force and motor units of small to intermediate size. Given these metrics, speech production falls into the category of a fine motor skill, similar in principle to playing a piano or violin.

The spatial precision just reviewed reflects only the *capabilities* or limits of the normal speech motor system. This precision may not be used in typical conversation and it can be shown to deteriorate with increases in speaking rate. As will be discussed later, speaking rate is a key variable in evaluating and treating individual dysarthric speakers.

Adaptive Control and Speech Motor Skill

> Adaptive control is loosely defined as any control that changes to meet changing needs....Thus, a well-designed adaptive system should continue to improve its performance based on past experience and readily adjust to new situations. For this reason, adaptive control is equated with learning.
>
> (Houk and Zev Rymer, 1981, p. 261)

Speech production meets the general requirements of a fine motor skill—that is, it (1) is performed with accuracy and speed, (2) demontrates motor flexibility in achieving goals, (3) is improved by practice, and (4) relegates all of this to automatic control, where consciousness is freed from the details of action plans (Wolff, 1979). As a motor skill, speech is goal-directed and afferent-guided. The goal is to produce the appropriate acoustic patterns via flexible motor *actions* that are formed and maintained by "auditory images." These auditory images, in turn, become yoked to the motor and somatoafferent patterns used to generate them (see Wolff's discussion of "perceptual motor ideas"). These "ideas" are highly similar to those of others (cf. Bernstein, 1967; Gurfinkel and Levik, 1979; Hardy, 1970; Ladefoged, DeClerk, Lundau, and Papcun, 1972; Mac-Neilage, 1970).

It is emphasized that these motor *actions* are not fixed movement routines or stored patterns of muscle contractions. The speaker's internal referent is what it feels like and sounds like tp produce certain speech movements and acoustics. Similarly, the "proficient violinist breaks a string while playing a recital but continues the performance without interruption by reprogramming the usual fingering and playing the required notes on different strings. The 'motor idea' controlling the musical performance does not prescribe a fixed relation between notes and finger movements, but enables the performer to generate functionally equivalent new finger sequences that will all preserve the musical passage" (Wolff, 1979). Comparable skills are evidenced in speech production (see review in Abbs and Cole, 1982).

Speech, in requiring adaptive control, represents one of the most advanced examples of selective access to muscles or pattern generators for the purpose of spontaneously creating novel motor acts—that is, those acts used to express a new thought of the speaker. Although it's reasonable to assume that humans are genetically predisposed to develop speech, they must be exposed to the appropriate sound patterns of a given language and undergo a reasonable period of sensorimotor learning in order to produce those sound patterns.

SPECULATIONS ABOUT NEURONAL MECHANISMS

Phylogeny and Ontogeny

In trying to understand how the human has developed the neuronal mechanisms for speech and language, we can look for clues in the phylogeny and ontogeny of the organism. The concept of the "triune brain" (a reticular to limbic to neocortical progression) is helpful in this regard (Brown, 1979; MacLean, 1970; Mysak, 1976). The human brain of modern people is not viewed as a simple layering-on of new to old brain but, rather, the elaboration and differentiation of each of the more primitive nervous systems, so that today's human is still very much in touch with, and influenced by, the reticular and limbic systems. Given this view, it is not surprising we have strong subcortical representations of speech, language, and thought. It is difficult to say whether the increased human capabilities are strictly a reflection of quantitative changes, as opposed to qualitative changes, in brain function. Nevertheless, there is little doubt that we possess the highest form of selective access to our motoneurons. This selective access is a key feature to our vocal tract and manual manipulative skills.

In ontogenetic development, myelinization proceeds from the brainstem outward, progressing both to the head and to the feet. Some cortical and subcortical regions develop earlier than others, and each regional development presumably is more complex in terms of the cognitive and sensorimotor skills it mediates. The rates of development even within a given cranial nucleus are differential and take place to serve the needs of the organism at particular points in time. For example, in the facial nucleus the lower portions develop more rapidly to serve the feeding functions required at birth, whereas the upper regions of this nucleus develop later in innervating the brown and other muscles of facial expression (Anokhin, 1974).

The infant also progresses through stages of development of reflexes, during which certain primitive and obligatory reflexes gradually disappear in the first 6 months, and other stereotyped patterns (e.g., righting and equilibrium reactions) appear in the second 6 months. The persistence of the primitive reflexes may interfere with the development of these reactions and any motor skills that depend on these reactions. It has been suggested that these primitive reflexes are placed under inhibitory control of the cerebrum and that they reappear with cerebral trauma (Capute, Shapiro, Palmer, Accardo, and Wachtel, 1981). A major theoretical issue is whether or not these reflexes are (1) *incorporated* into skilled motor acts, or (2) *inhibited,* or "gated-out" so as not to interfere with intended movements. Present data are sparse and provide no clear evidence for the incorporated or inhibited hypothesis. Capute and his associates suggest that of the seven primitive reflexes they have studied, only the tonic labyrinthine reflex significantly affects the oral-motor movements or positioning of normal infants. Obviously, the presence of strong normal or pathologic reflexes in the brain-injured will affect vocal tract movements. That is not to say that these reflexes are part of the speech motor control system.

Distributed Systems and Functions

Another important concept is that of *distributed* systems, especially in the neocortical system (see Mountcastle, 1978). This concept is highly similar to that of "functional systems" (see Anokhin, 1974). The concept here is that nuclei in different regions of the nervous system form interconnections to serve particular functions. Some functions share particular nuclei and pathways and not others. In addition, the "command neurons" for the different functions are located at different places in the nervous system. For example, breathing, sucking, chewing, and swallowing are thought to be driven by pacemaker neurons, or "pattern generators," located in the brainstem, whereas human speech motor control depends on more recently evolved neocortical structures.*

The concepts of distributed systems and functions gains some validity from clinical data. For example, selective damage to phylogenetically older parts of the cerebellum may affect walking and not talking. Conversely, walking can be preserved and a severe dysarthria result from damage to the neocerebellum. The distributed concepts also imply it is difficult, if not impossible, to destroy an entire function with a relatively small, localized lesion. Likewise, a localized lesion can disturb, at least in part, more than one function. The latter instances are most obvious at "summing points," or "final common pathways," in the nervous system—for example, at cortical or lower motoneurons where the nerve action potentials for more than one function are transmitted.

And finally, the distributed and distinctive nature of speech and language neural processes can be illustrated through electrical stimulation of different nuclei in the thalamus. Stimulation, even *within* the left ventrolateral nucleus, can either slow doen or speech up speech movements (Hassler, 1966; Mateer, 1978) and result in errors in naming or verbal

---

*Neocortical structures are not confined to cerebral cortex. They include at least the newer portions of the striatum, thalamus, and cerebellum (see review in Netsell, 1982).

memory (Ojemann and Ward, 1980). Lower stimulation current at these same sites accelerates memory processes, but not speech (Ojemann and Mateer, 1979).

Possible Roles of Afference

In addition to requiring hearing, the development of normal speech patterns is believed to rely on *somatoafference*. Somatoafference is defined here as receptor information from the sking, muscles, and joints concerning position and movement.

From Afference to Action to Higher Mental Functions. Many Russian investigators appear to assign primary importance to afferent mechanisms in developing and controlling skilled actions such as speech. These actions, in turn, are considered essential to the development of higher mental functions. For example, Luria (1980) says, "In the early stages relatively simple sensory processes, which are the foundation for higher mental functions, play a decisive role; during subsequent stages, when the higher mental functions are being formed, this leading role passes to the more complex system of connections that develop on the basis of speech, and these systems begin to determine the whole structure of the higher mental processes. For this reason, disturbance of the relatively elementary processes of sensory analysis and integration, necessary, for example, for the further development of speech, will be decisively important in early childhood, for it will cause the underdevelopment of all the functional formations for which it serves as a foundation (Luria, 1980, p. 35). Vygotsky formulated the following rule concerning the influence of a localized lesion at different stages of the development of a function: "In the early stages of ontogenesis, a lesion of a particular area of the cerebral cortex will predominantly affect a higher (that is, developmentally dependent upon it) center than that where the lesion is situated, whereas in the stage of a fully formed functional system, a lesion of the same area of the cortex will predominantly affect a lower center (that is, regulated by it)" (Luria, 1980, p. 35). Given the earlier discussion of the triune brain and its ontogenetic development, Vygotsky's rule should apply to the *distributed* speech motor system (i.e., brainstem and subcortical systems) as well.

Afferent Construction of Motor Acts. Grillner (1982) speculates that information from any relevant motor receptor system that is available may be utilized *at the time* a movement is planned to "construct" the motor command to be issued, so as to achieve an optimal pattern of activity. That is, the somatoafference is used by the child in constructing the original individual motor acts and in constructing a sequence of learned motor acts when expressing a novel thought through the speech motor system.

Grillner suggests that once speech motor acts have been learned, they are driven by "central programs," and these central programs use positive feedback as a means to construct the final motor output. This represents "a learned but subconscious type of pattern recognition of afferent information used to guide a central program" (Grillner, 1982, p. 221). With this concept, there is essentially instantaneous appraisal of the motoneurons generating the muscle forces concerning the state of the vocal tract. Earlier concerns that nervous system delays were too long for such fast modulations of motoneuron activity have been lessened by more recent theory and data (Abbs and Cole, 1982; Cole, 1981). Indeed, the neocortical system anatomy is such that both the cerebral and cerebellar cortices can be used in this afferent-efferent process.

Forward-Looking Control. Most of the concepts of feedforward and forward-looking control systems include some representation of the external world in the brain. For speech, some have suggested we develop a referent in terms of a vocal tract analogue (see review in Kent and Minifie, 1977). "If one accepts that the nervous system is probably developed so as to best do the job, the some ahead of time representation of movements is certainly expected" (Rack, 1981, p. 254). There may also be a provisional or initial command ("corollary discharge," "efference copy") that (1) accounts for the peripheral state of the vocal tract (position, velocity, plus, perhaps, acceleration), and (2) makes online changes in its controlling signal to the muscles. This internal revision of the controlling signal depends upon past experience as well as the present state of the vocal tract.

The embodiment of past experience is most often assigned to another construct of motor learning—that is, the "schema" (plural, "schemata").* In terms of speech motor control, schemata can be conceptualized as brain representations of what it sounds like and feels like to say or think a particular word or sentence.

Levels of Command Specificity

A key theoretical issue in motor control concerns the extent of detail that is specified at the input of the motor system under study. The range of possibilities includes the following: (1) Relative *gross* excitatory or inhibitory signals, or both, are hypothesized to activate subsequent mechanisms (for example, neural oscillators or pattern generators), which, in turn, carry out quasi-stereotyped motor actions. This option requires minimal detail from the central motor commands. The detail is in phasing the

---

*For discussion of schema in speech motor control, see Kent (1981) and Kent and Minifie (1977).

cycles of the lower level oscillators, but how this phrasing is learned, directed, or regulated for purposes of speech is not well formulated in the current explanations of the theory (see review in Kelso, 1981). (2) An intermediate level of command, or input specificity, calls for more *selective* activation of lower level mechanisms (for example, pattern generators), where the neural circuits used (for example, for walking) can be accessed at different points to yield independent movements (for example, flexing only the ankle or toe) (cf. Grillner, 1982). (3) At the level of extreme command specificity is the *direct-line* hypothesis, in which the cortical motoneurons have private and rather direct access to the lower motoneurons. This latter view regards cortical motoneurons as a summing point of (a) afferent and efferent information for the control of the muscles, and (b) the words selected to express the speaker's ideas. The essential problem to be solved is the most direct transform possible of the intended thought onto the controlling motoneurons. The controlling neurons have essentially instantaneous information about the present state or immediate future state of the vocal tract, or both. This may be sufficient updated and predictive information with which to modulate, *de novo*, the cortical motoneurons. This obviates the need for a provisional command to be revised and allows the "online" flexibility to begin vocalizing the thought and continue word selection even before the thought is complete (see Fry, 1966). It is also possible that this creative, "thoughtful" mode of talking engages brain mechanisms different from those used in rote speech, imitation, or in repeating nonsense syllables. The direct-line hypothesis relies minimally, if at all, on phylogenetically older mechanisms (e.g., brainstem pattern generators, or neural oscillators). For example, many speech patterns are immediately free of disorder with the remission of tremor. It seems as if the neural oscillators have superimposed a pathologic amplitude on otherwise normal speech movements. Once the amplitudes of these oscillations are reduced, the speech is perceived as normal. These clinical observations do not seem compatible with notions of *phasing* or *selectively activating* pattern generators or neural oscillators.

Each of the foregoing hypotheses emphasizes the availability and value of afferent information. None of these hypotheses has represented speech acts as a stringing together of "overlearned, stereotypic" motor patterns. However, the speech motor acts of a given language, once learned, are not infinitely flexible, but quasi-fixed, in that certain tightly coordinated movements cannot be broken up (except by neurologic lesion), and others are extremely difficult to learn or unlearn beyond a certain age.

Given its current sophistication, the human nervous system probably selects the best of its old and new mechanisms to formulate, initiate, and control speech motor acts.

A Continuum of Actions and Modes of Control

It has been suggested that *slow* movements can use limited servo assistance (e.g., by means of stretch reflexes), whereas rapid movements cannot (Rack, 1981). "For *rapid* movements the patterns of motoneuron activity must be computed and sent out without the benefit of immediate information about their effects" (Rack, p. 252). We speculated earlier that speech movements may be of moderate speed and thus benefit from a variety of modes of control. It may also be that different phases of speech movements are differentially controlled, and the same speech pattern (produced at faster speeds) may require shifts in the mode of control. Answers to some of these questions may come when discharge patterns of multiple motor units are studied for a variety of motor acts produced at varying speeds (e.g., comparing bilabial single motor units during three motor actions—such as nonspeech movements, saying "papapapapapa," and saying "Buy Bobby a puppy," in which each action is produced at slow, intermediate, and fast speeds). An experiment of similar principle has been proposed, in which nerve cell recordings at different loci within the monkey's nervous system would be compared for the activities of rhythmic chewing and controlled biting (Luschei and Goldberg, 1981). Burke's review (1981) of motor unit research provides some preliminary evidence that motoneurons are selectively activated for motor actions that are qualitatively different (i.e., under a different mode of control). Patterns of motoneuron recruitment may also differ as a function of speed of movement. Obviously, we would like answers to questions raised by these issues in considering what types of movements we ask dysarthric clients to make and what we conclude about their motor responses to our requests.

The Nature of Skilled Action Patterns. A final issue concerns the assumptions we make about the nature of skilled action patterns in general, and speech motor actions in particular. *If* there are encoding "units" smaller than words, what is their size and how, morphologically, are they represented? Grillner (1982), for example, speculates that speech motor actions are made up of "motor acts," of which "each motor act corresponds to a critical configuration of the oral cavity."

The Question of Unit Size. The available data offer little resolution to the question of "unit size" (see reviews in Kent and Minifie, 1977; MacNeilage, 1970). There are no data to show that units are of the size often practiced in speech therapy, that is, the phone (or phoneme), the consonant-vowel syllable, or other syllable forms. Also, in fractionating words or nonsense syllables into smaller, but potentially artificial, motor acts (e.g., in asking the client to first learn the motor act for *s*, then *ou*, and then *p*), we may be asking the client to learn separate motor acts that are not added together as they would be normally in saying the word "soup." Ideally, we would require practice of the requisite motor acts according to their true size as inputs to the speech motor systems. It also may be that the size of these input units changes during the acquisition of the language, although the *word* is an attractive candidate regardless of speaker age.

RELEVANCE TO THE DYSARTHRIAS

It is not possible in the space available to discuss in detail all of the ramifications of the foregoing for the clinical matters of the dysarthrias. As with many of the points covered in previous sections, many of these clinical implications clearly lie beyond the data available. As such, they are hypotheses to be tested.

Evaluating Speech Neural Mechanisms

Speech Versus Nonspeech Acts. Hixon and Hardy (1964) hypothesized that the most appropriate test of speech neural mechanisms was to observe vocal tract movements during the production of speech. The lumping of all vocal tract movements other than speech into the "nonspeech" category represents a semantic and conceptual hazard. The neuronal machinery or patterns of activation reponsible for sucking, chewing, swallowing, blowing, imitating orofacial movements, rapid alternating movements (with or without sound production), and isometric muscle contracts are hypothesized to be different from those used for speaking (see Dubner, Sessle, and Storey, 1978; Netsell, 1980). The nonspeech behaviors are often useful in determining the lesion(s)'s locus and general pathophysiologic consequence, but the activation of the speech neural mechanisms with *meaningful speech* may be the only valid test of function for the speech motor system.

There also is the concern that testing speech motor functions with sustained phonations, nonsense syllables, or "diadochokinetic rates" will yield results different from those gained with linguistically meaningful stimuli. For example, we saw a young boy recently who had substantial velopharyngeal opening when repeating /papapapapa/, but who achieved normal closure for words such as *puppy, puppy,* and *puffy.* It is a common clinical observation that velopharyngeal function during a sustained *ah* sound does not predict function during speech for the dysarthric individual. Miller and Hardy (1962) have shown marked differences in motor control of the tongue for speech and nonspeech movements in children with cerebral palsy. Even in normal speakers, laryngeal airflow during sustained vowels is generally lower than in consonant-vowel syllables (Smitheran and Hixon, 1981), and laryngeal resistance to airflow during non-sense syllables can be dramatically different from that recorded during meaningful words (Shaughnessy, Lotz, and Netsell, 1981).

Testing Component Function and Adaptive Control. The value of testing individual components of the speech mechanism is well known (cf. Abbs, Hunker, and Barlow, 1983; Hardy, 1967; Hixon, 1982; McNamara, 1983; Mysak, 1976; Netsell, 1976; Rosenbek and LaPointe, 1978). For example, holding the jaw in a fixed position, with a bite-block held between the teeth, is used to test independent functions of the lips and tongue. Better speech performance with the jaw fixed suggests that jaw abnormalities are contributing to the poor speech. Poorer speech with the jaw stabilized suggests the jaw is assisting (compensating for) the tongue or lips (or both) or biting on the block results in a spread of hyperactivity to the tongue or lips and affects their movements. Poorer performance with the jaw fixed also may indicate that the client has lost the adaptive control discussed earlier as motor equivalence.

An additional caution in interpreting component functions of the speech mechanism is that they may appear reasonably good on a component-by-component basis but look and sound quite poor collectively. Among the many possible reasons for this would be that the component analysis does not test the overall coordination of the speech mechanism. That is, in fractionating function of the whole system we have failed to test the coordination of the whole system. This concern is lessened by using meaningful speech stimuli that place primary demands on one component and minimal requirements on the others. For example, in testing lip function, use of the word "mom" or "mama" places emphasis on lip movements and lesser demands on the velopharynx, tongue, larynx, and respiratory system. A second reason for collective failure, or poor speech, with reasonably good individual components is that their summed small deficiencies added to a poor overall function. We recently saw a young man who had mild to moderate involvement of all components, no one of which would account for his generally unintelligible speech. A third hazard is that some components may appear severely involved in the presence of fairly adequate speech. Remaining adaptive control may be compensating for these more severe malfunctions, and treatment of them may be ill-advised. Many dysarthric clients have made adaptations to component malfunctions before coming to the clinic. The clinician must determine if these compensations are maladaptive. If so, they should be rehabilitated with regard to the pattern of deficits in the other components. If the compensations are not maladaptive and yield intelligible speech, the clinician may want to reinforce them and alter speaking rate or effort, or both, to further increase intelligibility.

Implications for Treatment

Several of the issues just raised bear directly on management decisions for the individual dysarthric client. Treatment considerations are outlined here for (1) restoring functions or skills that were acquired premorbidly, and (2) facilitating speech motor development in the brain-injured child. In general, the treatment approaches are conservative and eclectic. Since we lack data on the effectiveness of most individual and collective treatments, we can only intuit the appropriateness of a given procedure based on our knowledge of normal and abnormal mechanisms and clinical experience.

Restoration of the Speech Motor System. In cases of adult dysarthria, the two general goals are to (1) maximize the functional integrity of the musculoskeletal system (i.e., the vocal tract), and (2) require the nervous system to selectively engage its speech motor system.

Methods to optimize the expression of the speech motor system include (1) posturing to minimize the influence of pathologic reflexes (cf. Mysak, 1980); (2) other musculoskeletal alterations such as surgery, palatal lifts, bite-blocks, and abdominal binding; (3) orofacial stimulation and passive range of motion exercises to maintain sensorimotor and neuromuscular integrity, respectively; and (4) *minimal* strengthening exercises to maintain muscle mass. The methods under (3) and (4) are hypothesized to be of little value once some minimal speech movements can be elicited from the vocal tract component of interest. If the client can chew and swallow, this is probably sufficient activity to maintain at least muscle, nerve-muscle, and sensorimotor integrities for the neural mechanisms implicated in (3) and (4).

Several principles guide the selection of speech materials to be practiced. The starting points are taken from the client's available speech movements. Words are selected to preferentially activate muscles and muscle synergies over which the client has some control. Phonetic environments are chosen to facilitate the target movements. For example, work with nasal consonants in words could begin even if a substantial velopharyngeal problem was not yet managed. The most important achievement for the client is to reactivate the speech motor system and reexperience the motor output and somatoafference input associated with speech production. Speaking rate should be kept quite slow initially to allow as much movement-related afference as possible to be realized. Once the basic speech motor patterns have been restored, speaking rate can be adjusted to yield maximum intelligibility for the client.

Facilitating Development of the Speech Motor System. Methods to facilitate development of the speech motor system in a child with dysarthria would include the considerations already given for adults *plus* at least the following.

1. Speech motor practice should be with words that are developmentally appropriate. We see 6 year olds with unintelligible speech who appear to have the musculoskeletal and nervous systems of 3 year olds. The phonetic material should be geared to their developmental age.

2. Young children are still establishing the motor-afferent linkages (associations, "schemata") to be used as "central programs." Care should be taken in presenting phonetic stimulus materials to maximize early success as these children are forming perhaps the single most important mechanism of the speech motor system—that is, the internal associations of what it feels like to make the movements that generate the acoustics just produced.

3. In the absense of data to the contrary, it seems advantageous to use words as stimuli wherever possible. "One of the predictions from the schema theory is that the subject who receives variable practice develops a strong schema for motor production enabling him to more effectively generate *novel movements*. Now, since the schema refers to a *complex set of relations*, it would seem, for example, that in devising any training programme for schema development, it would make sense to know which of these relationships are weak, i.e., what are the *dimensions of control* which the subject currently cannot handle" (Whiting, 1980, p. 548; italics added). The most direct evidence we have of poorly controlled dimensions would seem to be the abnormalities in the speech movements. Elicitation of more correct movements with carefully selected word stimuli would seem most appropriate for facilitating the set of relationships between thoughts, words, movements, acoustics, and somatoafference.

4. A final consideration for children relates to the importance of speech in the development of higher mental functions. It would seem important that language and other cognitive therapies be coupled with speech motor practice. Whereas the practice of the best possible speech is important, its practice in a "thoughtful" environment should be even more helpful in establishing the "thought to speech" transformations that have formed a central theme in this presentation.

SUMMARY

Data from the past 10 to 15 years on the control of speech production and other motor systems reveal a fast, adaptive nervous system that appears capable of almost instantaneous construction of novel motor acts to express human thoughts through action. The precise neural mechanisms that are used to generate speech motor acts remain unknown for the most part. It is important clinically to be aware of alternative hypotheses about the neural basis of speech motor control when considering (1) what you ask the client to do during the speech examination, (2) how you interpret her or his behavior, and (3) the resultant decisions to be made regarding treatment.

ACKNOWLEDGMENTS

Raymond Kent provided helpful comments on an earlier version of this paper. This work was supported by the Boys Town National Institute for Communication Disorders in Children and the National Institutes of Health.

REFERENCES

Abbs, J., and Cole, K. (1982). Consideration of bulbar and suprabulbar efferent influences upon speech motor coordination. In S. Grillner, B. Lindblom, J. Lubker, and A. Persson (Eds.), *Speech motor control.* Elmsford, NY: Pergamon Press.

Abbs, J. H., Hunker, C. J., and Barlow, S. M. (1983). Differential speech motor subsystem impairments with suprabulbar lesions: Neurophysiological framework and supporting data. In W. R. Berry (Ed.), *Clinical dysarthria.* San Diego: College-Hill Press.

Anokhin, P. (1974). *Biology and neurophysiology of the conditioned reflex and its role in adaptive behavior.* Elmsford, NY: Pergamon Press.

Bernstein, N. (1967). *Coordination and regulation of movements.* Elmsford, NY: Pergamon Press.

Brooks, V. (1981). *Handbook of physiology: The nervous system.* Vol. 11, *Motor control.* Bethesda, MD: American Physiological Society.

Brown, J. (1979). Language representation in the brain. In H. D. Steklis and M. J. Raleigh (Eds.), *Neurobiology of social communication in primates: An evolutionary perspective.* New York: Academic Press.

Burke, R. (1981). Motor units. Anatomy, physiology, and functional organization. In V. Brooks (Ed.), *Handbook of physiology: The nervous system.* Vol. 11, *Motor control.* Bethesda, MD: American Physiological Society.

Capute, A., Shapiro, B., Palmer, F., Accardo, P., and Wachtel, R. (1981). Primitive reflexes: A factor in nonverbal language in early infancy. In R. Stark (Ed.), *Language behavior in infancy and early childhood.* New York: Elsevier/North-Holland.

Cole, K. (1981). *An empirical re-evaluation of minimum voluntary afferent-to-efferent pathway latencies in the orofacial system.* Unpublished master's thesis, University of Wisconsin.

Dubner, R., Sessle, B., and Storey, A. (1978). Peripheral components of motor control. In R. Dubner, B. Sessle, and A. Storey (Eds.), *The neural basis of oral and facial function.* New York: Plenum Press.

Fry, D. (1966). The control of speech and voice. In H. Kalmus (Ed.), *Regulation and control in living systems.* New York: John Wiley & Sons.

Grillner, S. (1982). Possible analogies in the control of innate motor acts and the production of sound in speech. In S. Grillner, B. Lindblom, J. Lubker, and A. Persson (Eds.), *Speech motor control.* Elmsford, NY: Pergamon Press.

Gurfinkel, V., and Levik, Y. S. (1979). Sensory complexes and sensorimotor organization. *Fiziologiya Cheloveka, 5*, 399–414.

Hardy, J. (1967). Suggestions for physiological research in dysarthria. *Cortex, 3*, 128–156.

Hardy, J. (1970). Development of neuromuscular systems underlying speech production. In *Speech and the dentofacial complex: The state of the art. ASHA Reports, 5*, 49–68.

Hassler, R. (1966). The thalamic regulation of muscle tone and the speed of movements. In D. Purpura and M. Yahr (Eds.), *The thalamus*. New York: Columbia University Press.

Hixon, T. (1982). Speech breathing kinematics and mechanism inferences therefrom. In S. Grillner, B. Lindblom, J. Lubker, and A. Persson (Eds.), *Speech motor control*. Elmsford, NY: Pergamon Press.

Hixon, T., and Hardy, J. (1964). Restricted motility of the speech articulators in cerebral palsy. *Journal of Speech and Hearing Disorders, 29*(3), 293–306.

Houk, J., and Zev Rymer, W. (1981). Neural control of muscle length and tension. In V. Brooks (Ed.), *Handbook of physiology: The nervous system. Vol. 11, Motor control*. Bethesda, MD: American Physiological Society.

Kelso, J. (1981). Contrasting perspectives on order and regulation in movement. In A. Baddeley and J. Long (Eds.), *Attention and performance IX*. Hillsdale, NJ: Lawrence Erlbaum.

Kent, R. (1981). Sensorimotor aspects of speech development. In R. Aslin, J. Alberts, and M. Peterson (Eds.), *Development of perception: Psychobiological perspectives* (Vol 1). New York: Academic Press.

Kent, R., and Minifie, F. (1977). Coarticulation in recent speech production models. *Journal of Phonetics, 5*, 115–133.

Kent, R., and Moll, K. (1975). Articulatory timing in selected consonant sequences. *Brain and Language, 2*, 304–323.

Ladefoged, P., DeClerk, J., Lindau, M., and Papcun, G. (1972). An auditory-motor theory of speech production. *UCLA Working Papers in Phonetics, 22*, 48–75.

Luria, A. (1980). *Higher cortical function in man*. New York: Basic Books.

Luschei, E., and Goldberg, L. (1981). Neural mechanisms of mandibular control: Mastication and voluntary biting. In V. Brooks (Ed.), *Handbook of physiology: The nervous system. Vol. 11, Motor control*. Bethesda, MD: American Physiological Society.

MacLean, P. (1970). The triune brain, emotion and scientific bias. In F. O. Schmitt (Ed.), *The neurosciences: Second study program*. New York: Rockefeller University Press.

MacNeilage, P. (1970). Motor control of serial ordering of speech. *Psychological Review, 77*, 181–196.

Mateer, K. (1978). Asymmetric effects of thalamic stimulation on rate of speech. *Neuropsychologica, 16*, 497–499.

Miller, J., and Hardy, J. (1962). Considerations in evaluating dysarthria. Paper presented at the meeting of the American Speech and Hearing Association, New York.

Mountcastle, V. (1978). An organizing principle for cerebral function: The unit module and the distributed system. In G. Edleman and V. Mountcastle (Eds.), *The mindful brain*. Cambridge, MA: MIT Press.

Mysak, E. (1976). *Pathologies of speech systems*. Baltimore: Williams and Wilkins.

Mysak, E. (1980). *Neurospeech therapy for the cerebral palsied: A neuroevolu-*

tional approach. New York: Teachers College Press.

Netsell, R. (1976). Physiological bases of dysarthria. Final report, Research Grant NS 09627. Bethesda, MD: National Institutes of Health.

Netsell, R. (1980). Speech motor control: Searching for specialized neural mechanisms. Paper presented to the Meeting on Speech Motor Control, Madison, WI.

Netsell, R. (1982). Speech motor control and selected neurologic disorders. In S. Grillner, B. Lindblom, J. Lubker, and A. Persson (Eds.) *Speech motor control*. Elmsford, NY: Pergamon Press.

Netsell, R., Kent, R., and Abbs, J. (1980). The organization and reorganization of speech movements. Paper presented at the meeting of the Society for Neurosciences, Cincinnati.

Ojemann, G., and Mateer, C. (1979). Cortical and subcortical organization of human communication: Evidence from stimulation studies. In H. D. Steklis and M. J. Raleigh (Eds.), *Communication in primates: An evolutionary perspective*. New York: Academic Press.

Ojemann, G., and Ward, A. (1980). Speech representation in ventrolateral thalamus. *Brain, 94,* 669–680.

Rack, P. (1981). Limitations of somatosensory feedback in control of posture and movements. In V. Brooks (Ed.), *Handbook of physiology: The nervous system. Vol. 11, Motor control*. Bethesda, MD: American Physiological Society.

Rosenbek, J., and LaPointe, L. (1978). The dysarthrias: Description, diagnosis and treatment. In D. Johns (Ed.), *Clinical management of neurogenic communication disorders*. Boston: Little, Brown and Co.

Shaughnessy, A., Lotz, W., and Netsell, R. (1981). Laryngeal resistance for syllable series and word productions. Paper presented at the meeting of the American Speech-Language-Hearing Association, Los Angeles.

Smitheran, J., and Hixon, T. (1981). A clinical method for estimating laryngeal airway resistance during vowel productions. *Journal of Speech and Hearing Disorders, 46,* 138–146.

Whiting, H. (1980). Dimensions of control in motor learning. In G. Stelmach and J. Requin (Eds.), *Tutorials in motor behavior*. New York: North-Holland Publishing Co.

Wolff, P. (1979). Theoretical issues in the development of motor skills. Symposium on Developmental Disabilities in the Pre-School Child, Johnson & Johnson Baby Products, Chicago.

Chapter 5

Physiological Studies
of Dysarthria and
Their Relevance to Treatment

This chapter is written primarily for the clinical researcher who must evaluate, and perhaps treat, the next dysarthric patient that enters the clinic. Designating the clinician a clinical researcher implies that understanding the speech production problems of each dysarthric individual is an "experiment," using the principles of the scientific method, including single-subject research design.

Most of the material presented here is drawn from five recent review articles that trace historical and current developments more thoroughly, albeit biasedly (Chapters 1 through 4 of this book and Netsell and Rosenbek, 1985). The interested reader is referred to these for literature references and the background for the hypotheses and points of view presented here.

The clinical specialists of the future in speech neuropathologies will benefit from research that has emerged in the past decade concerning speech motor control and its disorders. These more recent studies are applying modern approaches to motor control and clinical neurophysiological studies of the spinal nervous system to those of the cranial nervous system. Reviews of this work are found in Abbs and Cole (1982) and Abbs and Rosenbek (1985). For the present, and for the purposes of this chapter, I will attempt to present an intermediate position based on the assumptions that most current clinicians work primarily from perceptual (auditory and visual) analyses of dysarthric speech patterns, do not have a great deal of training in acoustic and physiologic analyses, and do not have the necessary instruments available in their clinic. In recognition of these clinical realities, the intermediate position will emphasize a conceptual framework for understanding and treating the dysarthrias. This framework focuses upon a physiological orientation to the dysarthrias, with one eye on behavioral tasks that yield reasonable hypotheses about the client under study and the other eye on the questions the clinician must ask the neuroscientists (anatomists, physiologists, and chemists) to obtain a better understanding of the biological determinants of that client's speech behavior.

THE CLINICIAN'S PROBLEM

Wendell Johnson (1946) posed three questions regarding problem-solving that the clinician can ask to understand the dysarthrias and any statements made by so-called authorities who presumably know something about the topic. The questions were "What do you mean?", "How do you know?", and "What difference does it make?" The question "What do you mean?" asks for the clearest possible definition of the term (word) or concept (groups of words) being expressed. "How do you know?" questions the bases (e.g., intuition, impression, data) and degree of confidence you have about your knowledge of the topic or issue in question. "What difference does it make?" assumes that, even if we are in reasonable agreement about *what* (definition) we are talking about and understand (knowledge) a great deal about it, to what extent would this make a difference in the way we think or behave?

To illustrate the value of Johnson's questions, consider the term *spastic dysphonia*. "What do you mean" by spastic dysphonia? What does the term "spastic" imply? Spasticity originally referred to a velocity-dependent, obligatory contraction of the muscle being stretched. More recently, it is used in a generic sense to refer to excess stiffness in muscle. Does using the term "dysphonia" imply that the problem is restricted to the larynx? Is "spastic dysphonia" neurogenic, psychogenic, or both? If neurogenic, is it implied that everyone who has spastic dysphonia has the same neuropathology?

Assuming for the moment that we agreed on the definition and homogeneity of neuropathology, "how do you know" the client in question has spastic dysphonia? Does he or she sound "spastic?" Does that mean that the voice sounds "strained," "hyperfunctional," "high pitched," or some combination? Are we in agreement as to what is meant by the terms "strained" and "hyperfunctional"? Regardless, the speech clinician hearing these voice characteristics would suspect a neuropathology and refer the client for a neurologic examination. What is to be learned from the neurologic examination? The neurologic examination might well appear normal overall, except for the "spastic"-sounding voice and heightened electromyographic (EMG) activity in the intrinsic laryngeal muscles. The heightened EMG activity could be neurogenic, compensatory activity, or some combination.

Even if we knew the patient had spastic dysphonia and had determined the neuropathogenesis, "what difference would it make"? Would the speech clinician, neurologist, or neurosurgeon treat the patient differently? The answer to this last question undoubtedly would be a resounding "yes"; the patient might receive optimal treatment if spastic dysphonia had a homogeneous pathogenesis and particular behavioral, pharmacological, or surgical procedures had been demonstrated to be the clear treatment of choice.

Johnson's three questions apply to almost all of the terminology and concepts in the dysarthrias, most of which have been borrowed from neurology. Ask a random selection of your colleagues "What do you mean?" and "How do you know?" when they use the following terms: "spasticity," "flaccidity," "athetosis," "ataxia," "dystonia," "dyskinesia," "tonicity," "strength," "muscle power," "timing," and "discoordination."

A PHYSIOLOGIC ORIENTATION

A physiologic orientation to the dysarthrias emphasizes that the individual's speech problem is one of motor control, secondary to a nervous system lesion or lesions. The clinician's task is to understand, to the extent possible, what has gone wrong with the speech mechanism of the next client seen in the clinic. To me this means we not only must examine the structural adequacy of the musculoskeletal system, we also must design tasks that will allow inferences to the neural mechanisms controlling the vocal tract movements. The design and interpretation of these tasks are at the heart of what is implied by the term "physiologic orientation" to understanding and treating the dysarthrias. Depending upon the experiences, training, and biases of the researchers involved, arguments are made that the perceptual, acoustic, and physiologic levels of speech analysis are the best way to improve our understanding of the dysarthrias. Ideally, a perceptual-acoustic-physiologic analysis should be made of each vocalization produced by each dysarthric speaker; but this, of course, currently is unrealistic. In this chapter the potential power, as well as shortcomings, of the physiologic analyses will be emphasized.

There is the possible illusion that, because physiologic studies are "closer to" the underlying neurophysiologic problem, they are our best chance to understand what has gone wrong with the nervous system. In my opinion, physiologic studies in isolation (that is, without concomitant measures of the perceptual or acoustic correlates) are uninterpretable. For example, if the physiologic data (such as movement and EMG patterns) from a selected dysarthric speaker and from a dyspraxic speaker were laid side by side, the physiologist could not discern what was "dysarthric" about the former patterns and what was "apraxic" about the latter patterns. In short, the physiology data must be tied to their acoustic-perceptual consequences. It is appreciated that most clinics do not have the necessary instruments to carry out physiologic examinations. Also, most clinicians have not yet been exposed to or trained in the use of such instruments and interpretation of the resulting data. It is to be hoped that this situation will be remedied over the years. Fortunately, a physiologic orientation does not require actual physiologic recording but rather an attitude—a set of ideas that allows physiologic interpretations and inferences to be made from controlled, systematic behavioral observations.

PHYSIOLOGIC STUDIES

A number of events in the mid- to late 1960s catalyzed the current interest in physiologic studies of the dysarthrias. First, there were major developments in instrumentation, including cineradiography, EMG electrodes, and strain-gauge transducers. (EMG is a technique for recording muscle action potentials [MAPs].) Even though the more appropriate term would be MAP electrodes or MAP patterns or activity, the current terminology usually refers to EMG electrodes, patterns, activity, and so on. Second, Hardy (1966) drew attention to the need for detailed physiologic studies of the dysarthrias. Third, Darley, Aronson, and Brown (1969a, b) reported that a given dysarthric speaker could be assigned to a particular dysarthric classification on the basis of the perceptual identification of a deviant set of speech and voice dimensions. More importantly, these investigators offered hypotheses about the underlying pathophysiology and neural lesions that determined the perceptual deviations for the six types, or classes, of dysarthria identified in their studies. These three events prompted the present author to begin perceptual physiologic studies of the dysarthrias (Netsell, 1971), from which developed the component analysis approach that is reviewed here.

THE MAYO STUDY IMPETUS

The Mayo Clinic perceptual study of the dysarthrias (see Darley et al., 1969a, 1969b, 1975) was an impetus to the physiology studies from the 1970s to the present for several reasons. First, the study drew attention to several forms of the disorder, and we now refer to "the dysarthrias." Unfortunately, some clinical researchers have adopted the Mayo classification of five forms of dysarthria (six forms when a mixed dysarthria exists) as the classification scheme for clinical and research purposes. The Mayo group identified the six forms primarily on the basis of the case load that was available in their clinic and did not intend, in this author's opinion, that this be regarded as the definitive clinical classification scheme for the dysarthrias. Second, the Mayo study encouraged clinical researchers to think in physiologic terms about the deviant speech and voice dimensions they heard in the client's speech patterns. Third, the six forms of dysarthria identified were drawn from seven neurologic entities (pseudobulbar palsy, bulbar palsy, Parkinson's disease, amyotrophic lateral sclerosis, cerebellar lesions, dystonia, and chorea). The implication was (and is) that the perceptual analysis has diagnostic (localizing) value and the types of dysarthria involve different "motor systems" or different nuclei or pathways used in speech motor control. The fourth impetus of the Mayo study was the challenge to researchers to test the neurological hypotheses generated by the perceptual analyses: "These conclusions may serve as hypotheses for more accurate physiologic and neurophysiologic measurements to further delineate the problems of dysarthria" (Darley et al., 1969a, p. 496).

Value of Physiologic Studies

Ostensibly, there are two good clinical reasons for physiologic studies of selected subgroups or forms of dysarthria: they may assist in the neurologic diagnosis and treatment, and they should provide more detail concerning the general speech motor deficits associated with particular neurologic entities. A third benefit of these studies is that often the pathophysiology reveals phenomena that must be interpreted against and accounted for by current hypotheses of normal speech motor control. An additional value of the pathophysiology studies reported to date is that they have pointed to a considerable range of speech motor deficits that can occur within a given dysarthric subgroup. For example, some parkinsonian patients speak too softly and slowly, whereas others speak too rapidly. Even though future research may reveal a unifying pathophysiology to explain these apparent disparate symptoms, the current research has reinforced the need to examine and account for individual differences within a given neurologic entity, whether or not that examination is in the traditional speech clinic or physiology laboratory.

Current Developments

To illustrate the value of physiology studies of the dysarthrias and the increasing sophistication of the instrumentation, data analysis, and interpretation, five investigations of parkinsonian dysarthria that appeared from 1972 to 1983 will be reviewed.

Leandersson, Meyerson, and Persson. Leandersson, Meyerson, and Persson (1972) studied 12 dysarthric patients with Parkinson's disease using needle electrodes in several facial muscles and the oscillographic record of the airborne acoustic signal to segment the speech sounds and interpret the EMG activity. (The interested reader may want to consult the Krival [1965] dissertation, which may have been the first EMG study of the dysarthrias.)

These investigators reported heightened EMG activity in antagonistic muscles during attempts at lip closing and opening for bilabial consonants as a prominent feature of all their parkinsonian subjects. They also noted that "the resting activity between utterances was markedly increased and often progressed to a sustained hypertonic background activity" (p. 271). In contrast, EMG activity in the facial muscles of their neurologically normal controls was minimal to absent during resting activity and markedly reduced, if not quiescent, in antagonist muscles during the bilabial movements. Leandersson and colleagues concluded that

> The hypertonic background activity, with no distinguishable articulatory activity superimposed, impedes the participation of these muscles in articulation, thereby reducing the number of muscles available for rapid articulatory movements. The uneven distribution of tonus disturbs the functional balance between the two muscle groups for lip-closing/opening. Hyperactivity of the lip openers may even counteract the function of the lip closers. (p. 276)

In further interpretation of their results, Leandersson and colleagues went on to remark:

> EMG studies of the limb muscles in Parkinsonism have shown that one of the most characteristic signs of the motor dysfunction is an impairment of the reciprocal innervation (Hoefer and Putnam, 1940; Schaltenbrand and Hufschmidt, 1957; Schneider, 1968). The current study demonstrates that the same type of disturbance may occur in the facial musculature. (p. 276)

And, in reference to the same point:

> Apparently there are characteristics which are common to the impairment of motor function of Parkinsonian limb and labial musculature. This is some-

what unexpected since limb muscles, being attached to the skeleton, perform joint movements, whereas labial muscles move soft tissues such as muscles and skin without necessarily having an attachment to bone. Furthermore, muscles of the lips differ from those of the limbs in that they contain very few or no muscle spindles (Kadanoff, 1956; Filogamo, quoted by Gandiglio and Fra, 1967). Yet, in spite of these important differences in functional anatomy, the type of disturbance in motor control seems to be similar in both kinds of muscle. This fact should be taken into consideration when discussing the neuromuscular basis for the motor symptoms in Parkinsonism. (p. 277)

The major conclusion of their research was that all untreated parkinsonian dysarthric patients presented a balanced hypertonia, and this hypertonia impaired their ability to produce rapid articulations. The presence of hypertonia was inferred from heightened EMG activity in almost all facial muscles. As previously noted, heightened EMG activity can occur for several reasons, including compensatory adjustments of the speaker. Also, movements of the articulators were not recorded and the hypothesis that rapid articulations were impaired was inferred from the duration of acoustic segments (that is, the voice signal). In the only data display for direct comparison of a normal and dysarthric subject, the acoustic duration of the [p] segments was nearly identical for the two subjects, and the lengthened dysarthric segments were for the surrounding vowels. Also, in the comparison of EMG and acoustic durations for a dysarthric subject before and after levodopa treatment, the authors point out dramatic reductions in the EMG activity following medication, but only the vowel durations are shortened and the [p] segments again appear similar in duration. The report by Leandersson and colleagues was qualitative in that they presented sample, or representative, data displays without actual measurements of EMG activity or acoustic segment durations. Evidence of heightened EMG activity in antagonistic muscles with concomitant slowing of movements would have strengthened their conclusions.

Marquardt. Marquardt (1973) recorded EMG activity from two muscles that elevate and depress the lower lip simultaneously with movements of the lower lip and jaw in four parkinsonian dysarthric patients and two normal control subjects. The most dramatic finding was that peak accelerations (corresponding to the maximum slope of the movement velocity) of lower lip elevatons for bilabial consonants in two of the parkinsonian subjects ranged from 200 to 800 cm/s^2 compared with the corresponding maxima of approximately 20 cm/s^2 in the neurologically normal control subjects. Given the speculations of Leandersson and colleagues concerning possible reductions in speed of articulation due to hypertonicity, Marquardt's observations of markedly increased velocity and acceleration of lower lip movement for two parkinsonian subjects stands in stark contrast. Marquardt's data pointed to extreme heterogeneity of speech symptoms in parkinsonian dysarthria and introduced at least a partial physical explanation for what Darley and colleagues had termed "short rushes of speech" that occurred in some, but not all, dysarthrias associated with Parkinson's disease.

Netsell, Daniel, and Celesia. Netsell, Daniel, and Celesia (1975) recorded surface EMG activity from the upper lip (musculus orbicularis oris superior), intraoral air pressure, and voice recordings from 22 dysarthric patients with Parkinson's disease and matched normal control subjects. They reported that half of the parkinsonian subjects demonstrated perceived "short rushes of speech" and in one data display showed evidence of successive EMG bursts for consecutive syllables that were produced at a rate equivalent to 13 syllables per second.

Given that the upper limit for normal repetition is fewer than 10 per second, the investigators concluded that the subject was in some neuromotor mode over which he had no immediate control. They also suggested that successive syllables appeared at shorter and shorter intervals and, perhaps, prematurely termed this phenomenon "acceleration of speech." In viewing these same data, Evarts (1981, personal communication) hypothesized that this may not be true acceleration of successive syllables, but rather a switch from a slower repetition rate to an abnormally fast, but uniform, rate. Netsell and colleagues also showed that this subject could produce essentially normal syllables at rates below 4 per second by following the simple instruction to speak with about twice the loudness of normal speech. I shall return to these issues later in discussion of the more recent study of Hunker and Abbs (1984).

The second hypothesis resulting from the study by Netsell and colleagues was that parkinsonian dysarthric patients exhibited "weakness" in developing the phasic muscle contractions for speech. Weakness was inferred from the low amplitude and short duration of EMG bursts from musculus orbicularis oris superior for lip closures associated with bilabial consonants. However, as with the data of Leandersson and colleagues, no quantitative analyses were reported and only one data display was presented. In noting the cinefluorographic study of Logemann, Blonsky, Fisher, and Boshes (1973), who reported that many parkinsonian dysarthric patients do not reach a requisite vocal tract configuration for a particular speech sound before moving on to the next sound in the sequence, Netsell and co-workers concluded that "(1) weakness in the control signals, rigidity, or the acceleration phenomenon could be the neuromuscular basis for this reduced range of movement, and (2) various combinations of these conditions are present in many parkinsonian individuals" (p. 175).

Hunker, Abbs, and Barlow. Hunker, Abbs, and Barlow (1982) provided the first quantitative evidence of hypertonia (increased stiffness) in the lip muscles of four subjects with Parkinson's disease. Separate measures of upper and lower lip stiffness were obtained as the subjects sat quietly and the experimenter displaced the lip to various levels with a cantilever beam that allowed measurement of the lip's opposing force to the displacement. EMG activity from both lips was recorded with hooked wires inserted into the muscles. On clinical examination, it was believed that two of the parkinsonian subjects (P1 and P2) had equal hypertonia (that is, increased resistance to the examiner's finger displacements) in both lips, whereas the other two subjects (P3 and P4) had greater hypertonia in the lower lip. The force-displacement data (see Figure 3 in the article by Hunker et al.) verified and quantified these impressions by showing that, at maximum lip displacements (6 mm), subjects P1 and P2 had stiffness values that were three- to fourfold greater than those of normal subjects in both lips, and subjects P3 and P4 had lower lip stiffness values approximately twice that of normal subjects, with upper lip stiffness being essentially normal. In a separate procedure, Hunker and associates recorded EMG and movement from the lips of their subjects during speech. The EMG patterns ressembled those of Leandersson and colleagues in that the upper and lower orbicularis oris muscles showed heightened EMG activity during lip-opening gestures, a time during which normal muscles are markedly reduced in their activity. In contrast to the normal subjects, all parkinsonian subjects' lip movements were slow and reduced in range of movement. More importantly, the reductions in range of movement for the upper or lower lip of a given dysarthric patient were related to their increased stiffness (hypertonia) measures obtained in the force-displacement procedure already described. The researchers hypothesized that the relationship of increased stiffness during passive displacements to the reduced range of motion and heightened EMG during speech provided "compelling evidence of a cause-effect relation between rigidity and some aspects of hypokinesia, especially reduced range of movement" (p. 752). Recognizing that the stiffness measures were made as the subjects sat quietly and that the heightened (antagonistic) EMG activity and reduced range of motion were recorded during speech, the investigators were appropriately cautious in suggesting their cause-effect relation was direct evidence that rigidity had been demonstrated to affect speech:

> Our observations confirm the suggestion that parkinsonism has an associated reduction in the range of orofacial movement or hypokinesia. However, without further investigation, it is not certain that reduced range of movement contributes in any simple manner to the so-called articulatory inaccuracies, unless the characteristic abnormal frication of stop conso-

nants is a perceptual and acoustic manifestation of articulatory under-shoot. (p. 754)

Hunker and Abbs. Hunker and Abbs (1984) recently reported a detailed study of orofacial tremor phenomena in eight parkinsonian patients and normal control subjects. Tremors were recorded under five conditions: (1) with the subjects sitting quietly "at rest"; (2) during "posturing," when the jaw was lowered to a position comparable to that for the vowel [ɑ]; (3) as the subjects generated isometric forces of labial closure; (4) during selected speech movments; and (5) during passive displacements of the lips "at rest" (as described in the study by Hunker and colleagues). The recorded variables of interest included positions and movements of the lips and jaw, passive and active forces of the lips, intramuscular EMG from selected perioral muscles, the airborne acoustic signal, and laryngeal vibrations with an accelerometer. A special feature of the data analyses was the spectral analysis of the EMG, force, and movement signals. The spectral analysis allowed identification of multiple peaks, corresponding to dominant and secondary tremor frequencies. Even though not all tasks and variables were recorded for each subject, the entire data set permitted a host of heretofore unreported observations of parkinsonian tremors in the orofacial system and hypotheses concerning their possible influences on speech motor control. Only selected findings are reviewed here, but the interested reader will find many other observations and hypotheses in studying the full report.

A major finding from the spectral analysis of the EMG, force, and movement signals was the presence of three spectral peaks, or tremor frequencies, occurring at three rather fixed intervals: 4.5, 9.0 and 13.5 Hz. Depending upon the subject's task, the relative amplitude of these peaks was shown to shift from one frequency to another in most of the parkinsonian subjects. By contrast, only the 9.0 Hz peak appeared in the normal data and only during the isometric force task. In citing the work of Freund and associates (Freund, 1982; Freund and Dietz, 1978), Hunker and Abbs point to several inferences regarding motor unit properties that might be drawn from the spectral analyses, including the observation that peak spectral frequency during the isometric force task correlates strongly with the fastest possible rate of voluntary movement. Interestingly, the 9.0 Hz peak in the normal data (actually shown as 8.4 Hz in Figure 6 of Hunker and Abbs) corresponds to the fastest possible rate of rapid, alternating speech movements. In contrast, the spectral peak of the parkinsonian subjects in the isometric force task was 4.6 Hz, and the authors hypothesize this as the approximate maximum rate of movement at which these subjects can control orofacial movement. Interestingly, when the patients were asked to produce a series of [pɑ] syllables "as rapidly but as accurately as possible, a rate of less than 5 Hz was always selected." When asked to exceed rates of 5 Hz, "labial movements became markedly reduced in range and an acceleration or hastening pattern was discernible." Even when syllables were produced at slow rates, an "action tremor" was superimposed on the lip movements and spectral peaks were observed at 4.5 and 9.0 Hz in both lips and jaw. Even though Hunker and Abbs presented no spectral displays during the patient's rapid speech (that is, above 5 Hz), it is tempting to speculate that 9.0 Hz (and possibly 13.5 Hz) peaks would have become dominant and contributory to the uncontrollably fast movements. Recall that the patient reported by Netsell and colleagues produced "indistinct syllables" at rates approximating 13 Hz and, when instructed to speak louder or with more effort, produced totally acceptable syllables at a rate of about 6 Hz. It may be that parkinsonian patients with substantial tremor avoid syllable rates that coincide with the spectral peaks, and, during attempts to speak faster, the syllable rates are "drawn to" and become "phase locked" with the spectral peaks of 4.5, 9.0, and 13.5 Hz. This would support the hypothesis of Evarts (1981, personal communication), previously mentioned, that these patients are not truly "accelerating" (producing successive syllables at faster and faster rates), but rather shifting quickly to fast (but quasi-fixed) rates that may be shown to coincide with one of the three dominant spectral peaks. In studying single-motor unit control of parkinsonian patients (in the biceps and first dorsal interosseous muscles), Petajan and Jarcho (1975) noted that units recruited with more than minimal muscle contractions often tend to fire in small groups at tremor frequencies.

Summing Up

As a group, the studies just reviewed demonstrate a chronology that has markedly increased our understanding of the pathophysiology of speech in Parkinson's disease. This understanding, in turn, has direct relevance to strategies for treating the speech disorders of these individuals. Whereas most perceptual analyses and earlier acoustic-physiologic studies considered tremor to be present on occasion, but not contributory to the speech problem, there is now reason to believe that tremor phenomena may be a prime determinant for many of the speech manifestations of Parkinson's disease. Recent treatments have emphasized delayed auditory feedback (Hanson and Metter, 1983) and speaking with increased loudness (Rubow and Swift, 1985). Both of these procedures resulted in the patients speaking at slower rates and with greater effort. It is tempting to speculate that the improved speech was produced at syllable rates of less than 5 Hz and that the pathologic tremor frequencies were avoided. On an even more optimistic note, Rubow and Swift report that their patient was able to transfer the clinically improved speech to the "real world" by wearing a portable feedback device that signaled undesirable reductions in vocal intensity.

A Call for Single-Subject Research

The studies of dysarthria subgroups to date have demonstrated general physiologic characteristics that are distinctive in a given subgroup and have pointed to marked individual differences, in terms of both the presence of particular distinctive characteristics and their differential severity in orofacial muscle groups (see also Barlow, 1984; Barlow and Abbs, 1983). These individual differences represent fertile ground for the use of single-subject experiments, especially in those subjects who are variable in their speech output. Stronger cause-effect statements should be possible by contrasting the perceptual-acoustic-physiologic correlates of the individual's poorer speech with those of his or her better speech.

RELEVANCE TO TREATMENT

The points of relevance in the discussed orientation and review to the treatment of individuals with dysarthria are obvious and numerous; each individual with dysarthria requires (1) a physiologic interpretation of their deviant speech and voice dimensions; (2) a speech mechanism examination that tests for differential involvement of the vocal tract components; (3) a tailor-made treatment program that encompasses the examination results and prognosis; (4) a careful documentation of the treatment effects; and (5) systematic reevaluations to monitor long-term changes in neurologic status and speaking ability.

Physiologic Interpretation

A physiologic interpretation of the dysarthric patient's speech patterns is drawn from the neurologic diagnosis and associated neurophysiologic testing and from speech mechanism examination results. It is simply insufficient and uninformative to say that the individual's speech is unintelligible and that he or she needs speech therapy. Hypotheses must be developed and tested as to "why" the speech is abnormal. For example, rather than simply recording on a phonetic chart that the client cannot make [k] or [g] sounds, the clinician would infer that the (1) hypoglossal nerve, (2) hypoglossal nuclei, (3) bulbar connectivities, or (4) suprabulbar pathways controlling posterior tongue movements were damaged. Information from the neurologic examination would then be used to infer the locus and nature of the neuropathologic disease. Unfortunately, the current state of the neurologic examination (including neurophysiologic testing and neuroimaging techniques) is best suited for problems of the spinal-motor system (as already mentioned). The choice of treatments (such as as pharmacologic, prosthetic, surgical, and behavioral) would be developed from the behavioral ("physiologic") and neurologic information. The speech clinician's role, as I see it, is fourfold: (1) provide the best possible description of the neuromotor control problem in speech; (2) provide the most appropriate behavioral therapy; (3) advise medical and dental colleagues regarding the clinical and research literature concerning effects of various treatments; and (4) document changes in speech motor control during and following the various forms of treatment.

SPEECH-MECHANISM EXAMINATION

Figure 5–1 is a useful diagram to summarize the results of the speech-mechanism examination. It requires the clinicians to make their "best guess" as to the severity of involvement in the various vocal tract com-

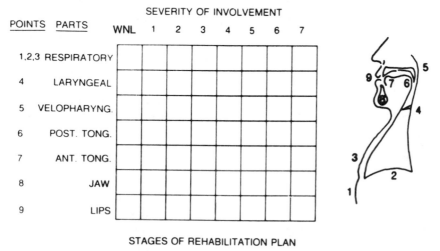

Figure 5–1. Rating form for severity of involvement of the vocal tract components and space for sequencing the goals and methods of the treatment program. WNL: within normal limits; 1: minimal involvement; 7: profound involvement.

ponents. Ideally, the clinician would be able to specify with certainty (1) which components are involved, (2) the relative severity of component involvement, (3) the contribution of each component to the aberrant speech, and (4) the neuropathologic bases of the involvement. Our current ability to achieve this ideal is technologically limited, but, conceptually, each of these four issues should be addressed, regardless of the clinician's sophistication and the availability of instruments. An overview of the approach to the speech-mechanism examination and its use in treatment planning is presented elsewhere (Netsell and Daniel, 1979; Netsell and Rosenbek, 1985; Rosenbek and LaPointe, 1978). The recent case study of Seif and Netsell (1984) illustrates the power of this approach even when instrumentation is not available.

Tailor-Made Treatments

Most of the dysarthric individuals for whom the physiologic approach is most appropriate have unintelligible speech at the initial examination, but they are capable of some vocal tract movements upon request. Our goal is to help them to be intelligible talkers, who use oral language as their primary means of communication. Augmentative communication aids often are necessary or useful in the initial and intermediate stages of treatment (see review in Linebaugh, Baird, Baird, and Armour, 1983).

Selecting and Sequencing Treatment Goals

The profile of vocal tract involvement is critical in selecting and sequencing the treatment goals. Several case studies now are available that illustrate different profiles and the rationale used in selecting and sequencing treatments, and these will not be reviewed here (Lybolt, Netsell, and Farrage, 1982; MacNamara, 1983; Netsell and Daniel, 1979; Rosenbek, 1984; Netsell and Rosenbek, 1985; Rubow, Rosenbek, Collins, and Celesia, 1984; Seif and Netsell, 1984; Shaughnessy, Netsell, and Farrage, 1983).

In general, we are quite aggressive in pursuing the goal of intelligible speech and very reluctant to abandon that goal, regardless of neurologic diagnosis. Our decision to pursue intelligible speech as a goal is based mostly on the individual's prognosis. Key factors in the prognosis include the patient's past and present neurologic involvement of the speech mechanism, response to previous therapy and our "diagnostic treatments," premorbid and current cognitive function, premorbid and projected personality and environment, and chronologic age (Rosenbek and Netsell, 1984).

Documentation and Reevaluation

It is critical to build on the modest beginning of published case studies that document the effect or lack of effect of given treatments with given dysarthric individuals. Single-subject designs provide the format, but clinicians must provide the skill in developing and carrying out the treatment scheme. Reevaluations of patients over a number of years also are critical to the evolution of our diagnostic, prognostic, and treatment skills. Even treatments that have been used for some time and have been shown to be effective in the short-term have not been subjected to long-term analysis. For example, prosthetic or surgical management of the velopharynx has been used with neurologic patients in this country for at least 25 years, and, yet, a recent survey of 374 cases revealed that fewer than 10 percent of these individuals were followed beyond two years (Lotz and Netsell, 1984).

UNANSWERED QUESTIONS

Basically, all the questions raised in this chapter and the extant literature are "unanswered" in that we need to know a great deal more about normal speech motor control, its development, and its disorders. Concerning Wendell Johnson's three questions posed early in this article, our answer to the third ("What difference does it make?") is that critical reading of the literature, and clinical practice around some variant of a physiologic orientation can make a big difference to the effectiveness of treatment with numerous dysarthric clients. Better clarification of terms and concepts ("What do you mean?") should lead to more insightful experiments of the mechanisms involved ("How do you know?"). Interdisciplinary teams of basic and applied researchers from the neurosciences, communication disorders, and related medical specialties seem to be prerequisites to approach these problems on a scale similar to that which has developed for the auditory system and its disorders.

Fortunately, most dysarthric individuals seen in the clinic experience improvement in their speech. Given that healing in the nervous system can be a long-term process, it often is difficult (if not impossible) to determine the contributions of various forms of treatment. The use of single-subject designs often, but not always, helps verify a treatment effect. Even the injured brain continues to "learn" and "relearn," and differentiating these processes from a treatment effect per se can be problematic, especially when the natural healing processes, learning and relearning functions, and treatment effects are interactive.

Perhaps the clearest evidence that how we think and what we know about the dysarthrias can yield more effective treatment comes from improvements in those individuals who have plateaued or failed to become intelligible with earlier treatments and become intelligible following treatment with the physiologic orientation described in this chapter (Lybolt et al., 1982; Netsell and Daniel, 1979; Rubow et al., 1984; Seif and Netsell, 1984). Nevertheless, the current form of this orientation is primitive in most respects, and its revisions (from the data and insights of basic and clinical researchers) should yield an even more powerful tool.

ACKNOWLEDGMENTS

The author's research and preparation of this manuscript were supported by the Boys Town National Institute and grants from the National Institutes of Health (NINCDS). I thank Ms. Carole Dugan for her usual excellence in manuscript preparation.

REFERENCES

Abbs, J.H., and Cole, K.J. (1982). Consideration of bulbar and suprabulbar afferent influences upon speech motor coordination and programming. In S. Grillner, A. Persson, B. Lindblom, and J. Lubker (Eds.), *Speech motor control*. Oxford: Pergamon Press, pp. 159–186.

Abbs, J. H., and Rosenbek, J. C. (1985). Some motor control perspectives of apraxia of speech and dysarthria. In J. Costello (Ed.), *Speech disorders in adults: Recent advances*. San Diego: College-Hill Press.

Barlow, S. (1984). *Orofacial subsystem force control in dysarthria*. Presented at the Annual Clinical Dysarthria Conference, Tucson, AZ.

Barlow, S. M., and Abbs, J. H. (1983). Force transducers for the evaluation of labial, lingual and mandibular motor impairments. *Journal of Speech and Hearing Research, 26*, 616–621.

Darley, F., Aronson, A., and Brown, J. (1969a). Differential diagnostic patterns of dysarthria. *Journal of Speech and Hearing Research, 12*, 246–269.

Darley, F., Aronson, A., and Brown, J. (1969b). Clusters of deviant speech dimensions in dysarthria. *Journal of Speech and Hearing Research, 12*, 462–496.

Darley, F., Aronson, F., and Brown, J. (1975). *Motor speech disorders*. Philadelphia: W. B. Saunders Co.

Freund, H.-J. (1982). Pathophysiological basis of some voluntary motor disorders. In B. Petterson and W. Zev Rymer (Chairs), *International Conference on the Neurophysiological Basis of Motor Disorders*. Chicago: Rehabilitation Institute of Chicago.

Freund, H.-J., and Dietz, V. (1978). The relationship between physiological and pathological tremor. In J. E. Desmedt (Ed.), *Physiological tremor, pathological tremor and clonus*. Basel: S. Karger, pp. 66-89.

Gandiglio, G., and Fra, L. (1967). Further observations on facial reflexes. *Journal of Neurological Sciences, 5*, 273.

Hanson, W.R., and Metter, E.J. (1983). DAF speech rate modification in Parkinson's disease: A report of two cases. In W.R. Berry (Ed.), *Clinical dysarthria*. San Diego: College-Hill Press.

Hardy, J. (1966). Suggestions for physiological research in dysarthria. *Cortex, 3*, 123–137.

Hoefer, P., and Putnam, T. (1940). Action potentials of muscles in spastic conditions. *Archives of Neurology, 43*, 704.

Hunker, C. J., and Abbs, J. H. (1984). Physiological analyses of parkinsonian tremor in the orofacial system. In M.R. McNeil, J.C. Rosenbek, and A.E. Aronson (Eds.), *The dysarthrias: Physiology, acoustics, perception, management*. San Diego: College-Hill Press, pp. 69-100.

Hunker, C.J., Abbs, J.H., and Barlow, S.M. (1982). The relationship between parkinsonian rigidity and hypokinesia in the orofacial system: A quantitative analysis. *Neurology* (NY), *32*, 749–754.

Johnson, W. (1946). *People in quandaries*. New York: Harper & Row.

Kadanoff, D. (1956). Die sensiblen Nervenendigungen in der mimischen Muskulatur des Menschen. *Zeitschrift fur Mikroskopisch-Anatomische Forschung, 62*, 1.

Krival, M. (1965). An electromyographic study of the orbicularis oris muscle in speech of people with Parkinson's disease. Doctoral dissertation, University of Wisconsin. Ann Arbor, MI: University Microfilms.

Leandersson, R., Meyerson, B. A., and Persson, A. (1972). Lip muscle function in parkinsonian dysarthria. *Acta Otolaryngologica, 74*, 271–278.

Linebaugh, C. W., Baird, J. T., Baird, C. B., and Armour, R. M. (1983). Special considerations for the development of microcomputer-based augmentative communication systems. In W.R. Berry (Ed.), *Clinical dysarthria*. San Diego: College-Hill Press.

Logemann, J. A., Blonsky, E. R., Fisher, H. B., and Boshes, B. (1973). *A cineradiographic study of lingual function in Parkinson's disease.* Presented at the Annual Convention of the American Speech-Language-Hearing Association, Detroit.

Lotz, W., and Netsell, R. (1984) *Effects of velopharyngeal treatment for individuals with dysarthria: Follow-up data and research needs.* Paper presented at the Clinical Dysarthria Conference, Tucson, Arizona.

Lybolt, J., Netsell, R., and Farrage, J. (1982). *A bite-block prosthesis in the treatment of dysarthria.* Presented at the Annual Convention of the American Speech-Language-Hearing Association, Toronto, Ontario, Canada.

MacNamara, R. (1983). A conceptual holistic approach to dysarthria treatment. In W.R. Berry (Ed.), *Clinical dysarthria*. San Diego: College-Hill Press.

Marquardt, T. (1973). *Characteristics of speech production in Parkinson's disease: Electromyographic, structural movements, and aerodynamic measurements.* Doctoral dissertation, University of Washington, Seattle.

Netsell, R. (1971). Physiological bases of dysarthria (Research Grant NSO9627). Bethesda, MD: National Institutes of Health.

Netsell, R., and Daniel, B. (1979). Dysarthria in adults: Physiologic approach to rehabilitation. *Archives of Physical Medicine and Rehabilitation, 40*, 166–174.

Netsell, R., Daniel, B., and Celesia, G. (1975). Acceleration and weakness in parkinsonian dysarthria. *Journal of Speech and Hearing Disorders, 43*, 326–330.

Netsell, R., and Rosenbek, J. (1985). Understanding and treating the dysarthrias. In J. Darby (Ed.), *Speech and language evaluation in neurology: Adult disorders*. Orlando, FL: Grune & Stratton, Inc., pp. 363–392.

Petajan, J., and Jarcho, L. (1975). Motor unit control in Parkinson's disease and the influence of levodopa. *Neurology (Minneap.), 25,* 866–869.

Rosenbek, J.C. (1984). Treating the dysarthric speaker. In J. C. Rosenbek (Ed.), *Current views of dysarthria. Seminars in speech and language,* Vol. 5: 359–384.

Rosenbek, J., and LaPointe, L. (1978). The dysarthrias: Description, diagnosis, and treatment. In D. Johns (Ed.), *Clinical management of neurogenic communicative disorders.* Boston: Little, Brown & Co.

Rosenbek, J., and Netsell, R. (1984) *Predicting failure to recover from brain injury and/or respond to treatment.* Presented to the Clinical Dysarthria Conference, Tucson, AZ.

Rubow, R.T., Rosenbek, J.C., Collins, M.J., and Celesia, G.G. (1984). Reduction of hemifacial spasm and dysarthria following EMG feedback. *Journal of Speech and Hearing Disorders, 49,* 26–33.

Rubow, R., and Swift, E. (1985). Microcomputer-based wearable biofeedback device to improve treatment carryover in parkinsonian dysarthria. *Journal of Speech and Hearing Disorders, 50,* 178–185.

Schaltenbrand, G., and Hufschmidt, H. (1957). Myographische Analyse des Parkinsonsyndroms. *Proceedings of the International Congress of Neurological Sciences, 1,* 94.

Schneider, P. (1968). Quantitative analyse und mechanism der bradykinesie bei Parkinson-patienten. *Deutsche Zeitschrift fur Nervenheilkunde, 194,* 89.

Seif, M., and Netsell, R. (1984). *Restoration of speech production thirteen years post-trauma.* Paper presented at the Clinical Dysarthria Conference, Tucson, AZ.

Shaughnessy, A., Netsell, R., and Farrage, J. (1983). Treatment of a four-year old with a palatal lift prosthesis. In W.R. Berry (Ed.), *Clinical dysarthria.* San Diego: College-Hill Press.

Chapter 6

Treating the Dysarthrias

Ronald Netsell
John Rosenbek

As recently as 30 years ago, many, if not most, clinicians and researchers appeared to believe that speech treatments for dysarthric talkers were of limited or no value. A common attitude, still held by some, was that the patient's speech handicap would follow the natural course of neurologic recovery or degeneration. Beliefs are changing. With respect to head injury, the old adage that no additional recovery can be expected two years after the initial trauma has been dispelled by our observations of continuing speech improvement four to five years after the trauma. Research in neurosciences, normal and dysarthric speech production, and the management of single patients (Netsell and Daniel, 1979) and occasionally even groups of patients (Scott and Caird, 1983) has provided data demonstrating that many dysarthric speakers can learn to speak more intelligibly. Even those with degenerative diseases such as amyotrophic lateral sclerosis and multiple sclerosis, and those with severe, chronic deficits, can be helped by appropriate selection from the behavioral, instrumental, and prosthetic methods to be described.

Reprinted by permission of the publisher from *Speech and language evaluation in neurology: Adult disorders*, J. Darby (Ed.), pp. 363–392. Copyright 1985 by Grune & Stratton, Inc., Orlando, Florida.

Managing the dysarthrias requires more than a technician's skills because treatment is more than the conscientious application of one or more techniques. Speech, regardless of most adults' facility with it, is an exquisitely complicated business, and learning to use a dysarthric system may be more complicated still. Clinicians, therefore, need to understand relationships among cognitive, linguistic, and motor processes as well as the facts and hypotheses about normal and disordered motor speech performance. They also do best if their activities are guided by a conceptual approach to the disorder they are evaluating and treating.

PHYSIOLOGIC APPROACH

The conceptual approach to the dysarthrias that has been most influenced by modern data on the relationship of cognition, language, speech, and the process of normal and abnormal speaking is what we term the *physiologic approach*. The physiologic approach as featured in this chapter refers to a set of ideas, including a neurobiologic view of human speech and its response to injury, that are used to form hypotheses about the biologic and behavioral bases for each dysarthric talker's speech disorder (see review in Netsell, 1984a). The dysarthrias are speech disorders, distinctly different from language disorders (such as the aphasias) and cognitive disorders (such as the dementias). The dysarthrias, however, can coexist with these and other conditions, and dysarthric speech is influenced by a speaker's linguistic and cognitive abilities.

The aim of a physiologic evaluation is (1) to determine the severity and type of involvement in each of the speaker's *functional components*,* (2) to determine the presence and severity of coexisting linguistic and cognitive deficits and the interactions of the motor, linguistic, and cognitive processes, and (3) then select and order the therapeutic targets and methods using knowledge of normal and abnormal speech production. Perceptual ratings of deviant speech and voice dimensions have been used primarily in helping establish the neurologic diagnosis (Darley, Aronson, and Brown, 1975; Metter, 1985). The physiologic approach is focused more on the symptoms and neurologic signs as they are differentially manifested in the functional components. Clinical evaluation, as governed by the physiologic approach, will be described in just enough detail to make a lengthier discussion of appropriate treatment procedures interpretable.

---

*A functional component is defined as a structure (or set of structures) that work to generate or valve the speech airstream (Netsell and Daniel, 1979).

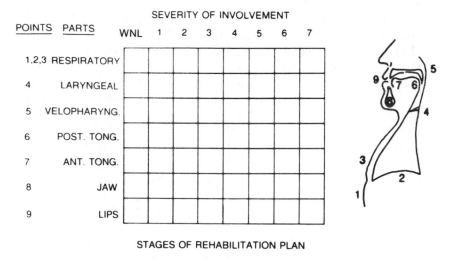

SEVERITY OF INVOLVEMENT

POINTS	PARTS	WNL	1	2	3	4	5	6	7
1,2,3	RESPIRATORY								
4	LARYNGEAL								
5	VELOPHARYNG.								
6	POST. TONG.								
7	ANT. TONG.								
8	JAW								
9	LIPS								

STAGES OF REHABILITATION PLAN

STAGE	PROBLEM(S)	PROCEDURE
1.		
2.		
3.		
ETC.		

Figure 6-1. Rating form for severity of involvement in each of the functional components and space for sequencing the goals and methods of the treatment program. WNL = within normal limits; 1 = minimal involvement; 7 = profound involvement. See text for details. (From Netsell, R., 1984b.) With permission.

Functional Components

Nine functional components primarily responsible for producing speech sounds (i.e., diaphragm, abdomen, rib cage, larynx, velopharynx, posterior tongue, anterior tongue, lips, and jaw) are shown in Figure 6–1.

Evaluation

Evaluation begins with testing of the functional components in isolation and in controlled combinations using speech and nonspeech stimuli, perceptual ratings, and (where available) instrumental measures.* One

---

*Instrumental measures refer to analog data generated by instruments that sense, transduce, and display any aspect of speech acoustics or physiology.

form of the perceptual evaluation appears in Rosenbek and LaPointe (1978). Perceptual evaluation is described in detail elsewhere (Darley et al., 1975; Metter, 1985). Netsell (1978) has written a description of some of the more available instruments and their use.

The perceptual data are first used to estimate the relative severity of each component's involvement and to generate hypotheses about why each component is impaired. The simplest measure of severity is a seven-point equal-appearing interval scale (Darley et al., 1975). A convenient form for displaying these relative severities appears in Figure 6–1. Instrumental evaluations such as (1) acoustic analysis, (2) aerodynamic testing, (3) fiberoptic and cinefluorographic videotaping, and (4) force, movement, and electromyographic (EMG) recordings also are useful in determining severity but are even more important in understanding why given speakers sound as they do.

Linguistic and cognitive deficits are determined by standard paper and pencil tests. These tests will not be described here. They are mentioned only as reminders that dysarthric talkers are more than talking machines and that dysarthric evaluation and treatment is more than testing and tuning the machinery.

Factors Influencing Treatment Decisions

Once a decision to treat has been made, clinicians need to decide which of a patient's functional components are to be treated and, if they are to be treated separately, in what order. They need to decide if treatment will be limited to a few days or will continue for a few weeks or months. They need to select and order one or more behavioral, instrumental, or prosthetic methods. *Behavioral* refers to traditional treatment methods in which a clinician provides a patient with counseling, education, an orderly progression of tasks to enhance performance, and knowledge of results. *Instrumental* treatments and methods for modifying posture have been arbitrarily excluded from the definition. *Prosthetic methods* refers to any physical alteration (including surgeries, medications, abdominal supports, palatal lifts, and bite-blocks) applied to or within the musculoskeletal or nervous system.

In addition to these general considerations, other factors can have a major or minimal influence on the treatment decisions made for a given patient. These factors include (1) the severity of neurologic insult, (2) underlying pathophysiology, (3) the medical status, (4) available methods and tools, (5) time available, and (6) the patient's need to communicate.

Severity

The selection and ordering of treatment methods is little influenced by the severity of neurologic involvement, unless the severity is rather specific to a given component. For example, many head injured patients show essentially no movement of the velopharynx during speech, and treatment of this component often is a necessary prerequisite to treatment of other components, such as the lips and tongue. With extreme hypernasality and loss of air pressure through the nose, many of these patients refrain from making lip and tongue movements because their speech remains unintelligible. These patients also illustrate that many dysarthric speech patterns are the combined result of the neurologic insult and their ability or inability to motorically compensate for the damage. The clinician must assess, to the extent possible, which aspects of motor involvement in each component are primary (neurologic sequelae) and secondary (voluntary or involuntary adjustments to or compensations for the damage).

A second principle to be followed in designing the treatment program is termed *peripheral dependencies*. This principle was well illustrated in the case study of Netsell and Daniel (1979) in which the head injured patient had major velopharyngeal and respiratory problems. Obviously, laryngeal and orofacial components are dependent on reasonable velopharyngeal and respiratory function for a sound (voice) source. Therefore, treatment was first directed at the velopharyngeal and respiratory problems. A corollary of the peripheral dependencies principle is to intervene against the component whose change will have the most general effect on the others.

Strict reliance on the severity criterion, however, may create a less than optimal treatment program. Sometimes beginning with a more mildly involved component gives the patient quick, motivating success that makes subsequent treatments more efficient.

Neuropathology

Obviously, the neuropathology responsible for the dysarthria will determine general neurologic signs associated with affected nuclei and their interconnections. Individuals with cerebellar involvement sound different from those with Parkinson's disease and have equally contrastive motor control problems. Even within a well-defined neurologic entity such as Parkinson's disease, however, the speech patterns and presumed underlying pathophysiology can be markedly different from individual to individual (see Netsell, Daniel, and Celesia, 1975). Because of this variability, the neurologic diagnosis per se is an insufficient basis on which to infer the physiologic basis of the individual's speech disorder and plan a treatment program. In addition, the presence of a given neurologic sign (e.g., spasticity) does not necessarily mean that it is fundamental, or perhaps even contributory, to the dysarthria (Barlow and Abbs, 1984). The onus is on the clinician to (1) evaluate the motor capability of each functional component as well as the component interactions in producing speech, (2) infer from the available data what neurologic signs are contributing to the component disorders, and (3) plan the treatment program accordingly. This is a highly inferential process at present, but the incorporation of clinical neurophysiology tests into speech examinations is ongoing and can be expected to strengthen such inferences in the near future (Abbs, personal communication, 1985; Netsell, Barlow, and Hunker, 1985).

Methods for treating physiologic dimensions directly are still being established and their effects on dysarthric speech are still being tested. Discoordination, resulting in a breakdown in integrated activities within one component or between two components, is often best treated by methods (to be described later) that enhance such integration rather than one focused on the function of individual components. Discoordination is most satisfactorily managed by behavioral methods. Thus, treatment (when successful) is often relatively brief. Whereas mild weaknesses can sometimes be influenced rather quickly (Netsell and Daniel, 1979), profound weakness often requires protracted treatment. This does not mean that very weak speakers are treatable only if bountiful resources are available. A variety of prosthetic and compensatory methods are possible, and in addition, alternative and augmentative systems using computers and other devices can be used (Linebaugh, Baird, Baird, and Armour, 1983). Abnormal tone also can be managed successfully with EMG biofeedback (Rubow, 1984; Rubow, Rosenbek, Collins, and Celesia, 1984).

Medical Status

The patient's disease (whether stable, progressive, or improving) and the availability and success of medical management also influence decisions about speech treatments. Managing a patient with stable or improving disease is as satisfactory to speech clinicians as to any other health professional, but degenerative disease such as amyotrophic lateral sclerosis does not necessarily obviate speech treatment. Indeed, selected methods such as the palatal lift have proved efficacious for such patients (Gonzalez and Aronson, 1970).

Speech treatments seem to work best for patients who also are responding simultaneously to other treatments. For example, the speaker with Parkinson's disease who is well controlled on medication does better in speech therapy than one who is having the "on-off effect" and other complications. Speech treatments, however, sometimes can succeed even when other treatments are unavailable or unsuccessful. Amyotrophic lateral sclerosis and multiple sclerosis are conditions for which medicine has no satisfactory treatment. Yet patients with these disorders sometimes do well with selected methodology described in the following section. Finally, speech clinicians can sometimes succeed even after once successful medical treatments have ceased to be successful. A voice amplifier, for example, may successfully amplify a parkinsonian patient's voice after medication has ceased to be maximally effective.

Available Methods and Tools

Most dysarthria treatment continues to be done with traditional behavioral methodology. Prosthetic and instrumental treatments, however, often are more efficacious as they lead to different decisions about how, what, and when to treat.

Instruments capable of providing biofeedback have proved especially useful. Such instruments make it easier to focus treatment on one functional component. Biofeedback treatments are most important in treating patients such as those described by Netsell and Daniel (1979) and by Seif and Netsell (1984). Indeed, both of the head injured patients described by these authors had previously failed to respond to behavioral treatment.

Time Available

Many conditions resulting in dysarthria do not require extended hospitalization. Patients with Parkinson's disease, for example, are most likely to be hospitalized only when the family needs a respite, the patient's medications are in need of titration, or the patient has other illnesses. Dysarthric talkers suffering from stroke or trauma may obtain adequate speech and language rehabilitation during the required hospital course for general physical rehabilitation. The clinical tendency in such cases is to manage several functional components simultaneously or to rely on relatively quick prosthetic management. Speechless or nearly totally unintelligible speakers and speakers with speech disorders of varying severity who want desperately to talk as normally as possible do come for therapy, and if resources are available to support it, protracted treatment can be successful. A combination of behavioral, prosthetic, and instrumental methods should be used with these severely handicapped patients. Behavioral methods usually are sufficient for highly motivated and somewhat more mildly affected dysarthric talkers.

Need to Communicate

Some dysarthric talkers reject speech treatment because oral communication is unimportant to them. In some cases, it is only fair to honor the patient's wishes. When the prognosis for speech restoration is reasonable, however, the clinician may need to insist on a contract with the patient for a trial period of treatment. Some dysarthric speakers may wish only to be intelligible to one or two familiar listeners. Clinicians may treat these patients using methods capable of effecting quick, but less than optimal, improvements. Other dysarthric talkers want to work toward the best possible speech. Probably no other influence on a clinician's decisions is as important as the patient's need to communicate.

METHODS OF TREATMENT

Dysarthric talkers can be treated with traditional behavioral methods, instrumentation (including biofeedback), postural adjustments, and prostheses. No one approach is a priori superior to any other. Given the present state of clinical science, treatment is tailored to each speaker regardless of the diagnostic category to which each has been assigned. In the treatment discussion to follow, methods will be emphasized rather than the criteria for choosing them. As an aid to organization, treatment methods for each of the functional components will be described first, followed by methods for managing several functional components simultaneously.

Respiratory System

The respiratory system is described here as consisting of the following: (1) muscles of inspiration and expiration, (2) lungs, (3) rib cage, (4) abdominal contents, and (5) sensory receptors and peripheral nerve innervation. Depending on posture and the demands of the speaking situation, the respiratory structures contribute differentially to generate and maintain a relatively constant subglottal air pressure (usually 5 to 10 cm H_2O). A secondary function of the respiratory system during speech is to generate brief increases in subglottal air pressure (50 to 100 ms in duration and roughly 0.5 to 1.5 cm H_2O in magnitude) during words that are strongly emphasized in a sentence. Hixon and colleagues have generated a data base and conceptual framework that represents our current understanding of speech respiration in normal and dysarthric speakers (see reviews in Hixon, 1973; Hixon, 1982; Putnam and Hixon, 1984).

Regarding functional components, we view the respiratory system in terms of the mechanics and muscle contractions acting on the rib cage, diaphragm, and abdomen (Hixon, 1973). Most conversational speech occurs in the midlung volume range (approximately 60 to 40 percent vital capacity). If a normal speaker reclines to the supine position, the effects of gravity add approximately 3 to 5 cm H_2O to the subglottal air pressure that would be generated in the upright posture in the midlung volume range (Hixon, 1973). Moving a patient with respiratory involvement to the supine position often is a useful clinical procedure since the subglottal air pressure increase can be sufficient for voice production in some cases.

As a clinical rule of thumb, we do not direct treatment to the respiratory system if the patient can generate a relatively steady ($\pm$ 1 cm H_2O) subglottal air pressure between 5 and 10 cm H_2O for 5 s (Netsell and Hixon, 1978). If there is a respiratory problem, most of the patients we have seen have reduced ability to reach these pressure levels. All of our treatments, therefore, have been aimed at increasing and maintaining subglottal air pressure. Of course, inefficient valving in the laryngeal, velopharyngeal, or orofacial systems will place greater demands on the respiratory system. Thus, it is critical to evaluate respiratory system function separately from the influences of the other functional components. Because we do not have the available instrumentation, we do not evaluate the component contributions of the rib cage, diaphragm, and abdomen. The necessary instruments and procedures for examining the respiratory components are described elsewhere (Hixon, 1983; Putnam and Hixon, 1984).

Inadequate overall loudness or loudness range and an irregular, inappropriate loudness change in connected speech may signal impairment of the respiratory system. However, hypoadduction or hyperadduction of the laryngeal airway and large velopharyngeal openings also can affect loudness. If clinical evaluation confirms a respiratory deficit, several treatment options are available.

Behavioral Treatment

Reduced loudness secondary to reduced subglottal air pressure often can be treated with behavioral methods. One of the simplest methods is to position the patient so that respiratory control is easiest. We ask dysarthric speakers if they notice differences in their loudness when lying down as compared with sitting up. Some speakers experience improved loudness in the supine or prone position. Increased loudness resulting from this postural adjustment is especially useful for speakers who are not ambulatory. Even when they are out of bed, they can be positioned in a wheelchair with an adjustable back that allows them to recline.

The clinician also can help some patients learn improved respiratory support without relying on instruments. The method involves helping the speaker monitor the amount of air inhaled and the evenness of each exhalation. Knowledge of results comes from listening to the loudness and from learning how to feel and see the result of being at the right size (i.e., from having the right volume of air available). Perceptible cues to the amount of inhalation are provided by outward movement of the abdomen or rib cage upon inhalation. The clinician can teach the patient what to watch for, and a patient with some arm control can monitor respiratory movements by placing a hand on the abdomen. How the air is used once inhaled will be signaled by the voice. A burst of loudness followed by quick decay means the inhaled air was released too quickly. Maintaining reasonable loudness over time usually means more normal control of exhalation, assuming there have been no major adjustments in laryngeal function. Speech stimuli can graduate from simple to increasingly complex.

Instrumental Treatment

A patient's subglottal air pressure can be increased by biofeedback with increased vocal loudness and loudness control as results. Instruments for providing the speaker with feedback about subglottal air pressure range from the simple and inexpensive to the sophisticated and more expensive. One of the simplest is a modified oral manometer (Netsell and Hixon, 1978). The tubing in this device is filled with colored water and mounted on centimeter graph paper. The patient blows into the tube, thus displacing the water. The amount of pressure is determined by noting the amount of water displacement in centimeters. The patient must be fitted with a leak tube during the procedure. The leak tube requires the patient to blow continuously. Without it, patients could merely generate a given pressure and then maintain it by holding their breath. The usual training procedure is to have patients generate progressively greater pressures (up to 8 to 10 cm H_2O) over longer periods of time (up to 5 to 8 s). Patients monitor the display for knowledge about performance. Once these targets are reached or patients have plateaued at some level, the instrument is systematically withdrawn. Patients begin speech drills, and auditory feedback about vocal loudness replaces visual feedback about subglottal air pressures.

Instead of providing feedback about pressure, some instruments provide feedback about vocal loudness. Rubow and Swift (1985) reported on a portable transducer that signals the wearer about loudness and computes the time the wearer spends talking at an appropriate loudness as determined by diagnostic testing. This device is especially promising because it extends clinical control outside the clinic and may reduce the risk of failure to carry over the clinical gains.

If all other methods fail, patients can be fitted with a portable voice amplifier. These devices, which work like any other amplifier system, require a microphone, amplifier, and power source. The microphone can be attached to the patient's glasses or even to a headband and positioned at the corner of the mouth. Greene and Watson (1968) reported on one patient's successful use of such an amplifier.

Prosthetic Management

The respiratory mechanism can sometimes be modified by prostheses. No standard prostheses exist and thus clinicians must create their own. The only requirement is that support be provided to the abdomen. One device is a paddle attached to a wheelchair that can be swung out when not in use and swung in and locked when the speaker prepares to talk (Rosenbek and LaPointe, 1978). Clinicians can determine this method's efficacy by using their own hands to brace the respiratory structures and encouraging each patient to speak. In this way, a clinician can experiment with amount of pressure and its timing during the respiratory cycle.

Laryngeal System

The laryngeal system is defined here to include the (1) intrinsic and extrinsic laryngeal muscles, (2) laryngeal cartilages and ligaments, (3) false, or ventricular, folds, (4) immediate subvocal fold space (rich in pressure and tactile receptors), and (5) sensory receptors and peripheral neural innervation.

Because of its multiple functions, the laryngeal system can be regarded as a microcosm of the entire speech mechanism. Its primary functions include (1) providing voicing through adduction of the true vocal folds; (2) generating silent periods (by means of abduction, as in / p /, / t /, and / k /) and other glottal openings for "noise sounds" (such as / h /); and (3) varying the fundamental frequency of vowel sounds, which the listener perceives as intonation or pitch variations of the voice. Fundamental frequency control is thought to be regulated primarily by cricothyroid muscle action. The adductory and abductory movements are controlled by the other intrinsic muscles.

Fiberoptic views of the glottal area show it to be almost continuously in movement during conversational speech; these dynamics qualify the laryngeal system as an articulator in the same way we regard the rapid movements of the velopharyngeal and orofacial structures. Static views of the larynx during sustained phonation (e.g., direct or indirect laryngoscopy) often miss cues to dysfunction that are revealed in the dynamics recorded with videofiberoptics. In a similar vein, laryngeal air flows during sustained vowel productions can be as much as three times different from those recorded during continuous speech (Netsell, Lotz, and Shaughnessy, 1984).

A secondary function of the laryngeal system during speech is the generation of loudness. The vocal folds must be moved medially and with sufficient medial compression to allow an audible vibratory pattern to occur. However, as mentioned previously, increases in loudness are thought to be regulated primarily by increases in subglottal air pressure, and the laryngeal muscles need only generate additional opposing forces to maintain the vibratory pattern (Hixon and Abbs, 1980). Future research undoubtedly will demonstrate the aforementioned account to be overly simplistic, but these are our current working hypotheses in evaluating and treating the laryngeal system.

The treatment of neurogenic laryngeal dysfunction, regardless of the methods used, usually is focused on one of two goals: (1) to aid the patient with hypoadduction to bring the folds medially, or (2) to help those with hyperadduction to reduce overclosure of the folds. Vocal tremor is relatively rare and some forms respond to medication (Aronson, 1980).

Behavioral Treatments

For the most part, we do very little in terms of directing behavioral treatments to the laryngeal system per se. If the patient is overadducting the folds, we know of no strictly behavioral method to modify this problem in the neurogenic patient. If the patient has any voice at all, our approach is to treat the other components first, and if a substantial voice problem remains, to (1) use contrastive stress drills (see section titled *Orofacial Treatments*) and (2) use sentence material that requires expressive (if not exaggerated) use of intonation.

If there is a major problem with the laryngeal system, it seems that the instrumental and prosthetic methods described later are prerequisites. Behavioral methods used to guide the patient in optimal pitch, loudness, and "tension" usage seem more efficacious following the instrumental or prosthetic treatments.

Instrumental Treatments

There are very few cases described in the literature concerning the value of biofeedback with neurogenic laryngeal disorders. Netsell and Daniel (1979) reported on a head trauma patient who was able to use visual feedback in reducing laryngeal air flow during speech. The flow reduction had no demonstrable effect on voice quality per se, but the authors were impressed that increased laryngeal control taxed the respiratory system less and provided the other structures with a more normal flow for articulation and resonance purposes.

Smitheran and Hixon (1981) described a patient with multiple cerebrovascular accidents (CVAs) and a "strained-strangled" voice that they attributed to increased laryngeal airway resistance (subglottal air pressure–laryngeal air flow). When the patient initiated speech at high lung volume levels, the resistance values decreased, as did the undesirable voice quality. The authors hypothesized that the use of high lung volumes caused a passive abduction of the vocal folds brought about by the tracheal tug associated with a lower diaphragm position. The patient was placed in a behavioral voice modification program and his response to treatment has yet to be reported. Nevertheless, these two patients point to the potential use of aerodynamic feedback with neurogenic hypoadduction and hyperadduction problems.

Even greater biofeedback potential may be found in future studies using videofiberoptics. This potential is illustrated in the case study of a young woman who developed dysphonia following strangulation (D'Antonio, Lotz, Chait, and Netsell, in press). Prior examination at another clinic indicated probable hysterical dysphonia with possible ventricular fold phonation. Behavioral therapy focused on increasing loudness, using the posttraumatic voice, and our opinion was sought because of the lack of improvement in voice function. The initial fiberoptic examination revealed ventricular fold phonation that allowed no view of the true folds. Subglottal air pressures were three times higher than normal (20 cm H_2O), laryngeal air flows were within the normal range (150 cc/s), and attempts to increase loudness exacerbated these problems. Using visual feedback of the videofiberoptic image during "inspiratory phonation," the true folds were visualized, and reduced mobility of the left arytenoid and vocal fold was observed. Using videofiberoptic feedback, the patient regained use of her true vocal folds, and the ventricular fold phonation remitted in four 20-minute treatment sessions. Her "true" voice was initially weak, but normal loudness was restored during treatment. At 20 weeks post treatment, her voice was essentially normal for conversational purposes, subglottal air pressure was normal (7 cm H_2O), and laryngeal air flow was only slightly elevated (250 cc/s). Our hypothesis was that the ventricular phonation was a subconscious, automatic compensation for the laryngeal damage and that any reference to psychogenesis was unnecessary, if not inappropriate, in this case.

Some individuals with a soft or weak voice (and sufficient subglottal air pressure) learn to increase their loudness using visual feedback (e.g., via an oscilloscope or voice light). Others with similar symptoms and normal respiratory function should benefit from the wearable feedback device of voice amplification (see Rubow and Swift, 1985).

Prosthetic Treatments

One of the most complete accounts of laryngeal reconstruction and related surgeries for voice restoration is by Hirano (1975). Unfortunately, it is only partially translated into English from the original Japanese. Hirano's work also is exemplary in that great care is taken to combine auditory–perceptual and instrumental evaluations (including stroboscopy and EMG) in both pretreatment and posttreatment examination of the laryngeal system.

In neurogenic dysphonias, most of the literature on surgical treatment focuses on (1) procedures to move one or both folds medially for phonation purposes (Hirano, 1975), and (2) recurrent laryngeal nerve (RLN) resection to paralyze one fold in cases of hyperadduction (Izdebski and Dedo, 1980). Regardless of the procedure used, one principle dominates: whenever possible, do not surgically destroy any portion of either vocal margin.

Resection of one RLN has become a popular procedure for relief of spastic dysphonia (Dedo and Shipp, 1980; Izdebski and Dedo, 1980). The procedure has been controversial in that others have reported a higher incidence of symptom recurrence than the 15 percent reported by Dedo and Shipp (e.g., Aronson and Desanto, 1983; Fritzell, Feuer, Haglund, Knutsson, and Schiratzki, 1982). The discrepancy may result from one of two factors or their combination: (1) definitions of spastic dysphonia vary and disorders so classified may be heterogeneous in etiology; and (2) criteria for patient selection may vary from clinic to clinic. Shipp (personal communication, 1984) reports that the San Francisco group (i.e., Dedo, Izdebski, and Shipp) is trying to clarify the situation by suggesting that spastic dysphonia be restricted in definition to hyperadduction of the folds (i.e., excessive medial compression). Excluded from this definition are tremor and neurologic signs implicating cerebellar, subcortical, or cortical involvement. The San Francisco group also suggests the following: (1) The neuropathology is brainstem in origin, with muscle and peripheral nerve being normal. (2) Symptoms recur only when the vocal folds develop sufficient medial compression to "retrigger" a pathologic laryngeal–brainstem interaction. (3) Recurrence is relieved by a second laser surgery that creates a longitudinal incision in the fold on the operated side, where the healing of the incision draws the fold laterally and out of "triggering" contact with the fold on the unoperated side. (4) Voice therapy is necessary in all cases to teach voice usage that will minimize redevelopment of hyperadduction by means of vocal fold contact. The typical result is a slightly breathy voice that is entirely functional and far superior to the original spastic dysphonia (Shipp, personal communication, 1984).

Unilateral vocal fold paralysis generally responds well to Teflon* injections (see Fritzell, Hallen, and Sundberg, 1974). Reabsorbable gelatin powder often is used as a trial to predict the results of the Teflon implants. Hirano (Wilson, personal communication, 1984) has developed a new procedure for patients with unilateral paralysis by inserting a cartilaginous wedge through a surgically created "window" in the thyroid lamina. The wedge is pushed medially until contact with the normal fold induces phonation. Parkinsonian patients considering cryogenic lesions of the ventrolateral (VL) thalamus for relief of rigidity or tremor below the neck should be advised that bilateral VL surgery can result in dysarthria, with

---

*Polytef Paste for Injection. Mentor Division, Codman and Shurtleff, Inc., Randolph, MA.

reduced vocal loudness as an especially intractable problem (Cooper, 1969).

Hixon (personal communication, 1964) suggested the electrolarynx might be a useful diagnostic tool when coordination of the respiratory and laryngeal systems with the orofacial and velopharyngeal systems was in question. The electrolarynx also may be useful as a treatment device when other methods have failed.

Velopharyngeal System

The velopharyngeal system is defined here as (1) the muscles of the soft palate (levator palatini and uvulae), (2) other muscles and structures of the upper pharynx, and (3) the sensory receptors and peripheral neural innervation that contribute to varying the size of the velopharyngeal (VP) orifice. Multiview cinefluroscopy and nasoendoscopic recordings of the velopharynx during speech show that normal and handicapped speakers use various combinations of these structures in closing or attempting to close the VP orifice (Croft, Shprintzen, and Rakoff, 1981; Glaser, Skolnick, McWilliams, and Shprintzen, 1979; Skolnick, McCall, and Barnes, 1973). Even in normal speakers, anatomic and EMG studies show wide variations in the muscles available and muscles used for VP closure and opening (e.g., see reviews in Dickson and Dickson, 1982; Fritzell, 1979; Kuehn, 1979). The only consistent finding across subjects is that the levator palatini is the primary muscle used to close the velopharynx. The uvula muscle appears more important than thought previously (Azzam and Kuehn, 1977). Its contraction bulges the levator eminence and its absence or reduction is a cardinal sign of submucous cleft and a high incidence of VP incompetence (Lewin, Croft, and Shprintzen, 1980). Given the individual differences in VP anatomy, muscle action, and patterns of VP closure, it follows that instrumental observations are mandatory when considering prosthetic treatment of velopharyngeal incompetence (VPI). As with the laryngeal system, the VP system is dynamic and should be regarded as an articulator. In saying the word *pump*, the velopharynx must close for the first /p/, open for the /m/, and close rapidly (within 50 to 75 ms) for the final /p/. Failure to close at the proper time will result in the perception of words such as *bum* or *mum* rather than the intended word. Oral views of the velopharynx during sustained *ah* vowels can be misleading. Some dysarthric individuals do not move the velum during this task and yet show good VP closure during speech. Others show substantial velar movement in the *ah* test and significant VP dysfunction during speech.

VP dysfunction in the dysarthrias basically is one of two types: (1) constant opening, or (2) intermittent and inappropriate opening. VPI designates a VP dysfunction that contributes significantly to the speech disorder. When multiple functional components are involved, as usually is the case in the dysarthrias, the determination that a given severity of VP dysfunction constitutes VPI can be difficult. As a general clinical rule of thumb, we find that moderate dysfunction (a severity rating of 4 in Figure 6–1) results in a VPI that requires treatment.

Severe VPI (severity ratings of 6 to 7 in Figure 6–1) is obvious to the listener as extreme hypernasality in voiced sounds and nasal emissions on oral consonants (e.g., /p/, /t/, /k/, /s/). In these severe cases, if speech intelligibility is noticeably improved by pinching the nares shut and having the patient produce a sentence with only "oral" sounds (e.g., *Buy Bobby a puppy*), the clinician can be quite confident that a successful VP treatment would benefit the patient. At the other extreme (severity ratings of 1 to 2), treatment focused on the velopharynx per se usually is contraindicated.

It is the "grey area" of VP dysfunction (severity ratings of 3 to 5) that is problematic in the treatment decision. The decision to treat the velopharynx in this grey area is based on the following considerations: (1) the relative severity of involvement in the other functional components; (2) whether treatment of the velopharynx would enhance function in other components (e.g., tax the respiratory system less or "encourage" more movement from the orofacial structures); and (3) whether VP function would be improved by treating other components first (e.g., improving respiratory, laryngeal, or orofacial functions), or simply having the patient speak more slowly and with greater effort.

Behavioral Treatment

Behavioral treatment of mild and some cases of moderate VP dysfunction often is effective (see section titled *All Components Simultaneously*). Also, some patients speak with a relatively closed mouth and this directs more air through the velopharynx. Speech exercises that emphasize more jaw opening and increased lip and tongue movements can decrease the negative perceptual impact of the mild–moderate VP dysfunction. As mentioned previously, speaking more slowly and with greater effort can increase both the orofacial and VP movements. One of our patients demonstrated dystonic movements of the lips, jaw, tongue, and velopharynx. VP dysfunction was intermittent and rated as moderate. Because the jaw appeared much more involved and contributory to the aberrant movements, we chose to treat it first. Using a bite-block prosthesis, the jaw was immobilized, lip and tongue movements were more normal, and a marked increase in intelligibility was noted (Lybolt, Netsell, and Farrage, 1982). In this case, the improved speech was so great that direct treatment of the VP dysfunction was unnecessary.

Our experience is that treatments involving blowing, gagging, suck-ing, and so forth, are ineffective in developing or restoring VP function for speech in dysarthric individuals. It may be, however, that certain dys-arthric patients would benefit from a procedure that involves the pairing of VP closure during blowing or whistling with vowel phonation in an oper-ant training program (see Shprintzen, McCall and Skolnick, 1975).

Instrumental Treatment

Biofeedback may be useful in helping individuals with dysarthria regain VP function. Collins, Rubow, Rosenbek, and Gracco (1981) used nasal air flow feedback with one dysarthric patient and reported success in the clinic setting. Two subjects with VPI but without a history of neuro-logic disease used visual feedback of the velopharynx with an oral panen-doscope (Shelton, Beaumont, Trier, and Furr, 1978). Both patients im-proved their VP function and speech. Generalization of these treatment effects outside of the clinic, however, was not demonstrated. With recent improvements in flexible fiberscopes inserted nasally, visual feedback training may be viable with selected dysarthric speakers prior to consider-ing more invasive prosthetic treatments. Those with less than severe VPI might be especially good candidates. If the patient could achieve closure with visual feedback, trials without visual feedback and reliance on audi-tory feedback and "muscle sense" should be introduced (see Rubow, 1984; Shelton et al., 1978). The reason we are optimistic that such biofeed-back treatments could be effective with certain dysarthric patients is that biofeedback and transfer of training of speech and other motor skills have been demonstrated with brain injured individuals (see reviews in Bach-y-Rita, 1980; Rubow, 1984).

Prosthetic Treatments

Even though prosthetic treatments are the most invasive and, theo-retically, should be considered only after all other treatments have failed, our preferred method of treating severe VPI in the dysarthrias is the palatal lift prosthesis. A recent survey of 415 cases showed that 50 percent experienced a 50 to 100 percent improvement in speech with a palatal lift (Lotz and Netsell, 1984). Almost 50 percent of these cases experienced dysarthria secondary to head injury. However, the survey also revealed that the long-term effects of palatal lift use have not been documented. Only 10 percent of the palatal lift cases in this series were followed beyond 2 years.

There are no generally agreed upon criteria as to who is a good can-didate for a palatal lift. The following clinical principle represents the criteria we have developed in dealing with more than 100 candidates. The best prognosis exists when there is (1) a large and constant VPI, (2) fair to good orofacial articulation, and (3) subglottal air pressure of 5 to 10 cm H_2O for a typical speech effort. At the other end of this continuum, the worst possible prognosis includes (1) a constant and large VPI, (2) poor orofacial articulation without much hope for improvement, and (3) subglottal air pressures under 4 cm H_2O. Note that a constant and large VPI is associated with both the best and poorest prognosis. Decisions to treat intermittent VPI are more difficult. In general, intermittent VPI associated with a moderate to severe dystonia (or athetosis) in the other functional components is a contraindication for prosthetic treatment of the velopharynx. LaVelle and Hardy (1979) report similar criteria based on more than 20 years of experience with this procedure. Details of the prosthesis construction are presented elsewhere (Schweiger, Netsell, and Sommerfeld, 1970).

The use of rhinomanometry has provided more quantitative measures of VPI (Isshiki, Honjow, and Morimoto, 1968; Netsell, 1969; Warren and DuBois, 1964). Based on their experience, Lotz and Netsell (1984) developed the following hypotheses regarding aerodynamic evaluations of VP dysfunction in the dysarthrias: (1) If nasal air flow on oral sounds is consistently above 200 cc/s, successful treatment of the velopharynx should increase speech intelligibility. (2) If nasal flows are in the range of 100/s, they do not have a major impact on intelligibility if intraoral air pressures for oral sounds are 5 to 10 cm H_2O and orofacial articulation is reasonable. (3) If intraoral air pressures are below 4 cm H_2O for oral sounds, nasal flows of 100 cc/s can be clinically significant and treatment of the velopharynx may be necessary. The third hypothesis seems especially valid if orofacial articulation is poor. In these cases, treatment usually is directed first at improving the range and accuracy of orofacial articulation. We must emphasize, however, that these hypotheses are based on clinical impressions and a number of well-documented cases are needed in order to test their overall validity.

The construction, fitting, and use of the palatal lift is not without problems. Some patients, even with successful desensitization of a hyperactive gag reflex (Daniel, 1982), cannot tolerate the prosthesis. Others, with strong velar, palatoglossus, or pharyngeal contractions, cannot retain the device. An additional key consideration is the skill level of the prosthodontist and the motivation of the patient. Optimal fittings of some palatal lifts require up to 60 days. Perhaps because of their more conservative case selection, LaVelle and Hardy (1979) fit most of their lifts in one or two visits.

Other clinicians prefer to treat VPI in the dysarthrias with a pharyngeal flap (see Johns and Salyer, 1978). The Lotz and Netsell (1984) survey showed the pharyngeal flap surgery to yield "speech improvement" similar to that reported for the palatal lift. However, most of the surgical results were evaluated in terms of "reduced nasality and nasal emissions." Data are not yet available concerning the surgical impact on improvement in speech intelligibility. When considering pharyngeal flap surgery, the ideal precursor is a trial with a palatal lift (Johns and Salyer, 1978). An earlier report on pharyngeal flap surgery for six children with cerebral palsy yielded equivocal results (Hardy, Netsell, Schweiger, and Morris, 1969). Three children improved their speech skills following surgery; the three who did not improve were reported to have a general lack of motivation to improve speech, academic skills, or activities of daily living.

Regardless of the prosthetic treatment of choice, videotaping of the nasoendoscopic examination has become an indispensable tool for determining the individual's pretreatment VP closure pattern, designing the lift or flap to that pattern, and evaluating the posttreatment function of the velopharynx. We also use auditory–perceptual evaluations and rhinometry, as described earlier. As in individuals with cleft palate, pretreatment movement of the lateral pharyngeal walls appears to enhance the success of VP treatment in the neurologically impaired.

Finally, all patients should be carefully counseled that intensive speech therapy will be necessary following any prosthetic treatment. Many of our "failures" have occurred when patients expect immediate intelligibility increases following prosthetic treatment.

Orofacial System

The orofacial system is composed of the (1) maxilla, mandible, and teeth, (2) muscles of the lower face, (3) tongue, (4) mid- to lower pharynx, and (5) sensory receptors and peripheral neural innervation of these structures. These components coordinate with the respiratory, laryngeal, and VP components to modulate the exhaled breath stream and produce intelligible speech. When dysarthria was previously defined by others as an "articulation disorder," dysarthria treatment often began and ended with articulation training of the orofacial components. Many dysarthric talkers continue to need such training, but most often as only one part of a more extensive, integrated program.

Behavioral Treatment

Only the most severely dysarthric talkers are incapable of making at least some differentiated speech sounds. Most dysarthric talkers are intelligible at least a portion of the time and to at least some listeners. Most focused orofacial treatments, therefore, are practiced on the severely involved patient. Behavioral treatments for these cases may begin by encouraging the talker to make any kind of predictable lip, tongue, or jaw movements. When such movements are possible, most clinicians have speakers add voice and try to produce differentiated American English speech sounds. Because most dysarthric speakers know exactly what they want to say, clinicians can rely less on the methods of traditional articulation therapy that were created to teach children and more on methods created specifically for the dysarthric talkers.

The clinician must individualize phonetic material and word lists for each patient that both (1) improve existing movement capabilities in some structures and, (2) facilitate nonexisting or minimal movement in other structures. Knowledge of the normal requirements of movement and muscle actions is essential to customize the speech movement sequences that are requested from a given patient. In essence, each time the clinician asks the patient to say something, the clinician must know in advance the physiologic demands of the task and the physiologic capability of the speaker. These general principles can be realized by a combination of "differentiating movements" and "exaggerating movements."

Differentiating Movements. The phylogeny and ontogeny of speech production can be thought of as an evolving differentiation, or fractionation, of vocal tract movements. As normal speaking adults, we combine these differentiated movements as rapidly as possible to signal as many contrastive sounds of meaning to the listener in the shortest period of time. For example, the words "pea," "tea," and "key" are realized by making the initial movements with the lips, tongue tip, and posterior tongue, respectively. It is estimated that we generate approximately 13 to 14 sound contrasts of meaning each second (Lenneberg, 1967). The movements required to make the "p," "t," or "k" sounds, for example, take about one tenth of a second (or 100 ms). Normal children do not reach adult-like speech and accuracy (i.e., precision) in speaking until early adolescence (Kent, 1976). The development of vocalization in infants and speech in children can thus be viewed as progressive increases in the motoric complexity required for the sounds produced (i.e., differentiated and co-occurring movements) (Kent, 1976; Netsell, 1981). Knowledge of these processes is critical to constructing individualized articulation drills according to (1) the patient's age and neuropathology, (2) differential involvement of the orofacial structures, and (3) whether the disorder is congenital or acquired. Because most of our experience has been with acquired adult dysarthrias, the remainder of this discussion will focus on therapy principles and procedures for this group.

Carefully planned therapy should minimize patient frustration and maximize their feelings of making progress. Typically this is possible by constructing meaningful words that are within the patient's physiologic capability and introducing speech movement demands from structures that are involved. As an example, it is common to see head injury patients with reasonable lip and jaw movements, variable anterior tongue control, and little or no movements of the posterior tongue. Initial emphasis is placed on making accurate movements (for example, complete closure of the lips for the word "Mom"). Note here that the physiologic demands of this word are minimal. The velopharynx can be open throughout and the jaw can assist in the lip closure as well as the vowel production. Differentiating lip movements can follow by having the patient perform the "f" sound, whereby the lower lip makes light contact with the upper teeth and the upper lip does not participate. Lip movements can then be further refined (i.e., differentiated) by stabilizing the jaw with a bite-block (Netsell, 1985). A bite-block is dental impression material that is form-fitted to the patient's teeth to effectively hold the jaw in a fixed position. This forces the patient to make all lip and tongue movements without assistance from the jaw.

Similar physiologic principles can be followed in helping the patient restore differentiated tongue movements for vowels and combined vowels (i.e., diphthongs). For example, initially let the patient make the "ee" versus "a" (as in "cat") vowel contrast using the jaw. This requires only that the tongue be slightly bunched and positioned anteriorly. The important, reinforcing word "yeah" can then be produced by positioning the tongue and sliding the jaw downward while vocalizing. Increasing difficulty and demands for differentiated tongue movements can follow at the appropriate time by introducing the bite-block.

A final principle in differentiating movements is called *facilitation*. Simply stated, this means to elicit or reinforce one movement, making sure to have the vocal tract shaped to facilitate that movement. For example, if movement for the "t" sound is the goal, use the vowel "ee" (as in the words "eat" or "tea"). The tongue will be positioned anteriorly and high for the vowel to facilitate tongue contact with the hard palate for the "t" production.

To summarize the foregoing and reinforce the reader's understanding of the general principles, consider the increasing physiologic difficulty in saying the words "Mom," "cat," and "scratch," respectively. Obviously, with the head injured patient described earlier, the first goal would not be a request to say the sentence, "Scratch the cat, Mom."

Exaggerating Movements. At some point in most patients' treatment they must practice making exaggerated movements with the orofacial structures during speech. Some dysarthric individuals may need only this form of treatment. The intent of exaggerated movements is to encourage a full range and accuracy of movement and let the talker hear and feel the results of these movements. Exaggerated movements usually are made more slowly than those that eventually will characterize the speaker's optimal speaking rate. Several procedures can be used to encourage these movements. Simply speaking loudly is one procedure. Loud speech requires more overall effort, and, presumably, this increase in effort translates to increases in force of contraction in the orofacial muscles. A similar rationale underlies the procedure of having the speaker bear down against a solid surface while speaking. Some of the postural and prosthetic adjustments described for the other functional components also make existing orofacial movements more effective in shaping the sounds of speech. Increasing the size of the bite-block can be helpful in forcing exaggerated movements of tongue elevation and lip closures.

Once a speaker begins combining at least a few differentiated sounds, these can be combined into meaningful, useful utterances. The clinician's emphasis throughout should be on intelligibility rather than on fine precision. Most dysarthric speakers move rapidly toward a wide repertoire of sound and sound combinations. Once they have that repertoire, the clinician can begin a series of specialized treatments that alter rate and stress so that the talker's speech is as intelligible as possible. These methods will be described in a subsequent section on simultaneous treatment of several components.

Instrumental Treatment

EMG plays a significant role in orofacial treatment. EMG signals have been used to improve facial muscle function following anastomosis of the facial nerve to a portion of the accessory nerve (Booker, Rubow, and Coleman, 1969) or to the hypoglossal nerve (Daniel and Guitar, 1978). In both instances, traditional treatments, such as practicing in front of a mirror, were of limited or no value. Netsell and Daniel (1979) used EMG feedback to improve the lip strength of one head injured dysarthric talker. The relationship of muscle strengthening to speech improvement remains controversial, but most clinicians persist with some form of strengthening when moderate to severe weakness exists. Whereas some clinicians have used maximal and sustained muscle contractions as a basis for strengthening (Dworkin and Hartman, 1979; Netsell and Daniel, 1979), Barlow (1984) has shown that dysarthric adults with cerebral palsy have a primary deficit in generating the rapid and relatively small muscle forces used in speech. Many of Barlow's subjects could achieve essentially normal maximal forces in the lips, jaw, and tongue. Future treatments of orofacial structures focused on fine force control may prove more efficacious than those of sustained maximal force. Transducers are now available for this purpose (Barlow and Abbs, 1983) and visual displays of force provide precise, immediate feedback and quantification of change. Both are important for learning and for documentation of treatment progress.

The relationship of abnormal tone and speech adequacy remains an experimental issue also. Nevertheless, clinicians have modified tone in a variety of patients with generally palliative effects on speech. Netsell and Cleeland (1973) treated a 64 year old woman with Parkinson's disease and severe retraction of the upper lip. In addition to being a cosmetic problem, the lip retraction interfered with production of some speech sounds. Within six 20-minute treatment sessions, this patient quickly learned lip control in nonspeech activities and experienced improved but imperfect control during speech. Hand, Burns, and Ireland (1979) demonstrated a similar effect on the abnormal lip activity of a 56 year old woman with Parkinson's disease and prominent retraction of the corners of the mouth at rest and during speech.

Finley and colleagues (Finley, Niman, Standley, and Ender, 1976; Finley, Niman, Standley, and Wansley, 1977) treated the speech of 10 cerebral palsied, dysarthric children with EMG feedback from the frontalis musculature. Since EMG signals from the frontalis muscle were used, this treatment probably had a more widespread effect on each speaker's tone that did the programs focused specifically on lip musculature. Finley and colleagues reported that this management was generally successful. These studies are noteworthy because they were successful, and because the second study (Findley et al., 1977) was structured to the requirements of a single case design. This second report also illustrated how biofeedback and a system of rewards can be combined.

Prosthetic Treatment

A few prostheses have improved orofacial function. A jaw sling was used with the 55 year old survivor of a series of brainstem strokes that left him anarthric and unable to close his mouth. The sling allowed him to close his mouth and eating was easier even though speech was still impossible because of lip and tongue weakness. He could place the food at the back of his mouth and then flip it into the oropharynx with a toss of his head. The posterior part of the swallow was intact and he swallowed once the food entered the oropharnyx.

A bite-block to stabilize the jaw also may improve some dysarthric speakers' orofacial movements. Diagnostic testing with and without a bite-block is an easy way of measuring the potential therapeutic value of the procedure. Two cases have been reported in which orofacial movements improved in the bite-block condition (Barlow and Abbs, 1979; DePaul and Abbs, 1984; Lybolt, Netsell, and Farrage, 1982).

The bite-block sometimes works because it helps a speaker inhibit abnormal, involuntary movements. It helps other speakers by stabilizing the jaw so that its movements do not have to be coordinated simultaneously with those of the lips and tongue. It may fail for some talkers, especially with significant weakness, who use the jaw to aid tongue movement.

All Components Simultaneously

At some stage in most treatments of patients with dysarthria, a shift is made from an emphasis on individual components to an emphasis on the simultaneous coordinated activity of all functional components. Treatments may even begin here for all but the more severely involved or for those with inordinately severe involvement of only one or two of the functional components. Simultaneous treatment of all components usually focuses on rate and word stress changes.

Behavioral Treatment

Simply telling a speaker to slow down or be more animated and try harder usually is ineffective. Learning to change rhythm, stress, or intonation requires drill. With intensive drill of the proper exercises, patients can be successful and instruments will be unnecessary. At least two methods lend themselves to such drill.

Gestural Reorganization. Gestural reorganization (Luria, 1970; Rosenbek and LaPointe, 1978) involves the combination of speaking and gesturing. In its simplest form, the speaker accompanies each syllable or word of a practice utterance with a simple tapping movement (Wertz, LaPointe, and Rosenbek, 1984). Prior to combining the two, assessments should be made of the patient's ability to tap and the influence of tapping on the speech paired with it. If tapping while talking is helpful, the two can be practiced in combination, and the gesture can be faded or not as the patient's speech adequacy permits. Gestural reorganization may be an intermediate step between the use of delayed auditory feedback and the simple admonition to slow down.

Contrastive Stress Drill. The contrastive stress drill (Fairbanks, 1960) is a question and answer dialogue in which word stress is made to move systematically but naturally by the questions asked. The underlying idea, although it has never been confirmed experimentally to our knowledge, is that articulatory movements are enhanced by increased stress. Drill materials, then, are organized so that the speaker uses primary stress on the target word or words. If, for example, the dysarthric speaker is working on /st/ blends, words such as *stay* and *sty* could be placed in sentences like "I want to stay" and "This place is a sty." To elicit primary stress on *stay*, the clinician could ask, "You want to what?" and it could be elicited on *sty* with a question such as "Isn't this place spotless?" With instruction, explanation, and coaching, a variety of dysarthric patients quickly accept and learn the drill. For the occasional patient who has trouble, the clinician can model both questions and answers and provide a variety of other cues. If simple stress does not facilitate improved articulatory accuracy, the clinician can help the speaker to increase his or her pause time or make other changes in prosody to enhance the procedure's effect (see Rosenbek and LaPointe, 1978).

Instrumental Treatment

The simplest treatment for modifying rate and stress is the pacing board (Helm, 1979). The patient is taught to accompany speech with systematic movements along or around the pacing board. For example, the speaker could begin by touching a portion of the board on each syllable while counting from 1 to 10. For patients with sufficient control of one hand and arm, this gestural accompaniment may help the speaker slow rate and exaggerate stress differences, with improved intelligibility as a result.

Delayed auditory feedback (DAF) also can slow a dysarthric talker's rate and improve intelligibility. Anecdotal (Rosenbek and LaPointe, 1978) and controlled (Hanson and Metter, 1980, 1983) reports demonstrate that DAF can be effective with some dysarthric patients. Hanson and Metter (1980) reported on the therapeutic effects of a portable DAF for a patient with progressive supranuclear palsy. While under 100 ms of delay, the speaker's rate was slowed and speech was louder and more intelligible. This patient responded despite having a progressive disorder and a history of failure with traditional therapy. This same unit was subsequently used (Hanson and Metter, 1983) to treat two patients with Parkinson's disease. The only difference in these two patients' treatments was that 150 ms of delay rather than 100 ms was used. Both patients spoke better under DAF, and neither speaker was successful in controlling rate without the DAF. The authors conclude, "The increase in physiological effort associated with increased the loudness may somehow override or suppress a neural feedback circuit that is involved in the acceleration behavior" (p. 246).

Dysarthria rate also has been controlled by biofeedback. Berry and Goshorn (1983) reported that their patient with multiple cerebrovascular accidents (CVAs) learned to speak target utterances slowly enough so that an electronic signal representing the speaker utterance filled the screen of an oscilloscope. This patient is reported to have slowed his speech and increased intelligibility by lengthening his pause time or the time between words. Yorkston and Beukelman (1981) used oscilloscopic feedback to teach one ataxic talker to increase his pause time or silence between words and another to increase his articulation time. Both patients were successful. Caliguiri and Murry (1983) used the oscilloscope to provide three dysarthric speakers with information about word stress. Some speech improvement was reported for each patient, even though their diagnoses were (1) pseudobulbar palsy secondary to bilateral CVAs, (2) ataxic dysarthria secondary to cerebellar infarct, and (3) a mixed dysarthria secondary to a 34 year history of multiple sclerosis.

REFERENCES

Aronson, A. (1980). *Clinical voice disorders: An interdisciplinary approach.* New York: Thieme-Stratton.

Aronson, A. E., and DeSanto, L. W. (1983). Adductor spastic dysphonia: Three years after recurrent laryngeal nerve resection. *Laryngoscope, 93,* 1–8.

Azzam, N., and Kuehn, D. (1977). The morphology of musculus uvulae. *Cleft Palate Journal, 14,* 78–87.

Bach-y-Rita, P. (Ed.) (1980). *Recovery of function: Theoretical considerations for brain injury rehabilitation.* Baltimore: University Park Press.

Barlow, W. (1984). *Orofacial subsystem force control in dysarthria.* Presented at the Annual Clinical Dysarthria Conference, Tucson, AZ.

Barlow, S. M., and Abbs, J. H. (1979, November). *Transducers for evaluation of articulatory muscle strength.* Paper presented at the American Speech and Hearing Association, Atlanta, GA.

Barlow, S. M., and Abbs, J. H. (1983). Force transducers for the evaluation of labial, lingual and mandibular function in dysarthria. *Journal of Speech and Hearing Research, 26,* 616–621.

Barlow, S., and Abbs, J. (1984). Orofacial fine motor control impairments in congenital spasticity: Evidence against hypertonus-related performance deficits. *Neurology, 34,* 145–150.

Berry, W. R., and Goshorn, E. L. (1983). Immediate visual feedback in the treatment of ataxic dysarthria: A case study. In W. R. Berry (Ed.), *Clinical dysarthria.* San Diego: College-Hill Press.

Booker, H. E., Rubow, R. T., and Coleman, P. J. (1969). Simplified feedback in neuromuscular retraining: An automated approach using electromyographic signals. *Archives of Physical Medicine and Rehabilitation, 50,* 621–625.

Caliguiri, M. P., and Murry, T. (1983). The use of feedback to enhance prosodic control in dysarthria. In W. R. Berry (Ed.), *Clinical dysarthria.* San Diego: College-Hill Press.

Collins, M. J., Rubow, R. T., Rosenbek, J. C., and Gracco, K. (1981). *An instrumental approach to reduction of nasal emission in dysarthria.* Paper presented to the American Speech and Hearing Association National Convention, Los Angeles.

Cooper, I. (1969). *Involuntary movement disorders.* New York: Harper & Row.

Croft, C. B., Shprintzen, R. J., and Rakoff, S. J. (1981). Patterns of velopharyngeal valving in normal and cleft palate subjects: A multi-view videofluoroscopic and nasendoscopic study. *Laryngoscope, 91,* 265–271.

Daniel, B. (1982). A soft palate desensitization procedure for patients requiring a palatal lift prosthesis. *Journal of Prosthetic Dentistry, 48,* 565–566.

Daniel, B., and Guitar, B. (1978). EMG feedback and recovery of facial and speech gestures following neural anastomosis. *Journal of Speech and Hearing Disorders, 43,* 9–20.

D'Antonio, L., Lotz, W. K., Chait, D. and Netsell, R. (in press). A perceptual-physiologic approach to the evaluation and treatment of dysphonia. *Annals of Otology, Rhinology, and Laryngology.*

Darley, F. L., Aronson, A. R., and Brown, J. R. (1975). *Motor speech disorders.* Philadelphia: W. B. Saunders.

Dedo, H., and Shipp, T. (1980). *Spastic dysphonia.* San Diego: College-Hill Press.

DePaul, R., and Abbs, J. (1984). *A physiologic and acoustic analysis of the effect of a bite-block prosthesis in a spastic dysarthric.* Paper presented at the Clinical Dysarthria Conference, Tucson, AZ.

Dickson, D., and Dickson, W. (1982). *Anatomical and physiological bases of speech.* Boston: Little, Brown.

Dworkin, J. P., and Hartman, D. E. (1979). Progressive speech deterioration and dysphagia in amyotrophic lateral sclerosis: Case report. *Archives of Physical Medicine and Rehabilitation, 60,* 423–425.

Fairbanks, G. (1960). *Voice and articulation drillbook.* New York: Harper & Row.

Finley, W., Niman, C., Standley, J., and Ender, P. (1976). Frontal EMG-biofeedback training of athetoid cerebral-palsy patients. *Biofeedback and Self-Regulation, 1,* 169–182.

Finley, W., Niman, C., Standley, J., and Wansley, R. A. (1977). Electrophysiologic behavior modification of frontal EMG in cerebral-palsied children. *Biofeedback and Self-Regulation, 2,* 59–79.

Fritzell, B. (1979). Electromyography in the study of velopharyngeal function: A review. *Folia Phoniatrica, 31,* 193–202.

Fritzell, B., Feuer, E., Haglund, S., Knutsson, E., and Schriatzki, H. (1982). Experiences with recurrent laryngeal nerve section for spastic dysphonia. *Folia Phoniatrica, 34,* 160–167.

Fritzell, B., Hallen, O., and Sundberg, J. (1974). Evaluation of Teflon injection procedures for paralytic dysphonia. *Folia Phoniatrica, 26,* 414–421.

Glaser, E., Skolnick, M., McWilliams, B., and Shprintzen, R. (1979). The dynamics of Passavant's ridge in subjects with and without velopharyngeal insufficiency: A multi-view videofluoroscopic study. *Cleft Palate Journal, 16,* 24–33.

Gonzalez, J. B., and Aronson, A. E. (1970). Palatal lift prosthesis for treatment of anatomic and neurologic palatopharyngeal insufficiency. *Cleft Palate Journal, 7,* 91–104.

Greene, M. C. L., and Watson, B. (1968). The value of speech amplification in Parkinson's disease patients. *Folia Phoniatrica, 20,* 250–257.

Hand, C. R., Burns, M. O., and Ireland, E. (1979). Treatment of hypertonicity in muscles of lip retraction. *Biofeedback and Self-Regulation, 4,* 171–182.

Hanson, W. R., and Metter, E. J. (1980). DAF as instrumental treatment for dysarthria in progressive supranuclear palsy: A case report. *Journal of Speech and Hearing Disorders, 45,* 268–276.

Hanson, W. R., and Metter, E. J. (1983). DAF speech rate modification in Parkinson's disease: A report of two cases. In W. R. Berry (Ed.), *Clinical dysarthria.* San Diego: College-Hill Press.

Hardy, J., Netsell, R., Schweiger, J., and Morris, H. (1969). Management of velopharyngeal dysfunction in cerebral palsy. *Journal of Speech and Hearing Disorders, 34,* 123–137.

Helm, N. (1979). Management of palilalia with a pacing board. *Journal of Speech and Hearing Disorders, 44,* 350–353.

Hirano, M. (1975). Phonosurgery: Basic and clinical investigations. *Otologia, 21,* 239–442.

Hixon, T. (1973). Respiratory function in speech. In F. Minifie, T. Hixon, and F. Williams (Eds.), *Normal aspects of speech, hearing and language* (pp. 78–124). Englewood Cliffs, NJ: Prentice-Hall.

Hixon, T. (1982). Speech breathing kinematics and mechanism inferences therefrom. In S. Grillner, B. Lindblom, J. Lubker, and A. Persson (Eds.), *Speech motor control.* (pp. 75–93). New York: Pergamon.

Hixon, T., and Abbs, J. (1980). Normal speech production. In T. Hixon, L. Shriberg, and J. Saxmon (Eds.), *Introduction to communication disorders* (pp. 43–87). Englewood Cliffs, NJ: Prentice-Hall.

Isshiki, N., Honjow, I., and Morimoto, M. (1968). Effects of velopharyngeal incompetence upon speech. *Cleft Palate Journal, 5,* 297–310.

Izdebski, K., and Dedo, H. (1980). Spastic dysphonia. In J. Darby (Ed.), *Speech evaluation in medicine* (pp. 105–127). New York: Grune & Stratton.

Johns, D., and Salyer, K. (1978). Surgical and prosthetic management of neurogenic speech disorders. In D. Johns (Ed.), *Clinical management of neurogenic communicative disorders* (pp. 311–331). Boston: Little, Brown.

Kent, R. (1976). Anatomical and neuromuscular maturation of the speech mechanisms: Evidence from acoustic studies. *Journal of Speech and Hearing Research, 19,* 421–477.

Kuehn, D. (1979). Velopharyngeal anatomy and physiology in relation to speech production. *Ear, Nose, and Throat Journal, 58,* 316–321.

LaVelle, W. E., and Hardy, J. (1979). Palatal lift prosthesis for treatment of palatopharyngeal incompetence. *Journal of Prosthetic Dentistry, 42,* 308–315.

Lenneberg, E. (1967). *Biological foundations of language.* New York: John Wiley & Sons.

Lewin, M., Croft, C., and Shprintzen, R. (1980). Velopharyngeal insufficiency due to hypoplasia of the musculus uvulae and occult submucous cleft. *Plastic and Reconstructive Surgery, 65,* 585–591.

Linebaugh, C. W., Baird, O. T., Baird, C. B., and Armour, R. M. (1983). Special consideration for the development of microcomputer-based augmentative communication systems. In W. R. Berry (Ed.), *Clinical dysarthria.* San Diego: College-Hill Press.

Lotz, W., and Netsell, R. (1984). *Effects of velopharyngeal treatment for individuals with dysarthria: Follow-up data and research needs.* Paper presented at the Clinical Dysarthria Conference, Tucson, AZ.

Luria, A. R. (1970). *Traumatic aphasia: Its syndromes, psychology and treatment.* The Hague: Mouton.

Lybolt, J., Netsell, R., and Farrage, J. (1982). *A bite-block prosthesis in the treatment of dysarthria.* Paper presented at the American Speech and Hearing Association Convention, Toronto, Canada.

Metter, J. E. (1985). Motor speech production and assessment: Neurologic perspective. In J. Darby (Ed.), *Speech and language evaluation in neurology: Adult disorders* (pp. 343–362). Orlando: Grune & Stratton.

Netsell, R. (1969). Evaluation of velopharyngeal function in dysarthria. *Journal of Speech and Hearing Disorders, 34,* 113–122.

Netsell, R. (1978). Physiologic recording in the evaluation and rehabilitation of dysarthria. *Communicative Disorders: An Audio-Journal for Continuing Education.* New York: Grune & Stratton.

Netsell, R. (1981). The aquisition of speech motor control: A perspective with directions for research. In R. Stark (Ed.), *Language behavior in infancy and childhood* (pp. 127–156). New York: Elsevier-North Holland.

Netsell, R. (1983). Speech motor control: Theoretical issues with clinical impact. In W. R. Berry (Ed.), *Clinical dysarthria*. San Diego: College-Hill Press.

Netsell, R. (1984a). A neurobiologic view of the dysarthrias. In M. McNeil, J. Rosenbek, and A. Aronson (Eds.), *The dysarthrias: Physiology–acoustics–perception–management*. San Diego: College-Hill Press.

Netsell, R. (1984b). Physiologic studies of dysarthria and their relevance to treatment. In J. C. Rosenbek (Ed.), *Seminars in speech and language: Current views of dysarthria*. New York: Thieme-Stratton.

Netsell, R. (1985). Construction and use of a bite-block in evaluating and treating speech disorders. *Journal of Speech and Hearing Disorders, 50,* 103–106.

Netsell, R., Barlow, S., and Hunker, C. (1985). Omaha, NE: Boys Town National Institute, Human Communication Laboratories.

Netsell, R., and Cleeland, C. S. (1973). Modification of lip hypertonia in dysarthria using EMG feedback. *Journal of Speech and Hearing Disorders, 38,* 131–140.

Netsell, R., and Daniel, B. (1979). Dysarthria in adults: Physiologic approach to rehabilitation. *Archives of Physical Medicine and Rehabilitation, 60,* 502–508.

Netsell, R., Daniel, B., and Celesia G. (1975). Acceleration and weakness in Parkinsonian dysarthria. *Journal of Speech and Hearing Disorders, 40,* 166–174.

Netsell, R., and Hixon, T. J. (1978). A noninvasive method for clinically estimating subglottal air pressure. *Journal of Speech and Hearing Disorders, 43,* 326–330.

Netsell, R., Lotz, W., and Shaughnessy, A. (1984). Laryngeal aerodynamics associated with selected voice disorders. *American Journal of Otolaryngology, 5,* 397–403.

Putnam, A. H. B., and Hixon, T. J. (1984). Respiratory kinematics in speakers with motor neuron disease. In M. R. McNeil, J. C. Rosenbek, and A. E. Aronson (Eds.), *The dysarthrias: Physiology–acoustics–perception–management*. San Diego: College-Hill Press.

Rosenbek, J. C., and LaPointe, L. L. (1978). The dysarthrias: Description, diagnosis and treatment. In D. Johns (Ed.), *Clinical management of neurogenic communicative disorders* (pp. 251–310). Boston: Little, Brown.

Rubow, R. (1984). Role of feedback, reinforcement and compliance on training and transfer in biofeedback-based rehabilitation of motor speech disorders. In M. McNeil, J. Rosenbek, and A. Aronson (Eds.), *The dysarthrias: Physiology–acoustics–perception–management*. (pp. 207–230). San Diego: College-Hill Press.

Rubow, R. T., Rosenbek, J. C., Collins, M. J., and Celesia, G. G. (1984). Reduction of hemifacial spasm and dysarthria following EMG feedback. *Journal of Speech and Hearing Disorders, 49,* 26–33.

Rubow, R., and Swift, E. (1985). Microcomputer-based wearable biofeedback device to improve treatment carryover in parkinsonian dysarthria. *Journal of Speech and Hearing Disorders, 50,* 178–185.

Schweiger, J., Netsell, R., and Sommerfeld, R. (1970). Prosthetic management and speech improvement in individuals. *Journal of American Dental Association, 80,* 1348–1353.

Scott, S., and Caird, F. (1983). Speech therapy for Parkinson's disease. *Journal of Neurology, Neurosurgery and Psychiatry, 46,* 140–144.

Seif, M., and Netsell, R. (1984). *Restoration of speech production thirteen years posttrauma*. Paper presented at the Clinical Dysarthria Conference, Tucson, AZ.

Shelton, R., Beaumont, K., Trier, W., and Furr, M. (1978). Videoendoscopic feedback in training velopharyngeal closure. *Cleft Palate Journal, 15,* 6–12.

Shprintzen, R., McCall, G., and Skolnick, M. (1975). A new therapeutic technique for the treatment of velopharyngeal incompetence. *Journal of Speech and Hearing Disorders, 40,* 69–83.

Skolnick, M., McCall, G., and Barnes, M. (1973). The sphincteric mechanism of velopharyngeal closure. *Cleft Palate Journal, 10,* 286–305.

Smitheran, J., and Hixon, T. (1981). A clinical method for estimating laryngeal airway resistance during vowel production. *Journal of Speech and Hearing Disorders, 46,* 138–146.

Warren, D., and DuBois, A. (1964). A pressure-flow technique for measuring velopharyngeal orifice area during continuous speech. *Cleft Palate Journal, 1,* 52–71.

Wertz, R. T., LaPointe, L. L., and Rosenbek, J. C. (1984). *Apraxia of speech in adults: The disorder and its management.* New York: Grune & Stratton.

Yorkston, K. M., and Beukelman, D. R. (1981). Ataxic dysarthria: Treatment sequences based on intelligibility and prosodic considerations. *Journal of Speech and Hearing Disorders, 46,* 398–404.

AUTHOR INDEX

Abbas, P., 47
Abbs, J.H., 4, 5, 6, 8, 23, 35, 37, 38, 42, 43, 44, 45, 47, 57, 62, 64, 65, 72, 79, 89, 90, 91, 95, 99, 105, 112, 113, 114, 116, 128, 134, 144, 145
Accardo, P., 10, 13, 93
Allen, G., 35
Anokhin, P., 9, 11, 18, 92, 93
Armour, R.M., 78, 118, 128
Aronson, A., 34, 39, 41, 42, 44, 46, 108, 109, 134
Aronson, A.E., 56, 57, 71, 72, 79, 128, 136
Aronson, A.R., 124, 126
Azzam, N., 137

Bach-y-Rita, P., 38, 39, 54, 75, 139
Baird, C.B., 78, 118, 128
Baird, J.T., 78, 118, 128
Baken, R., 13
Barlow, S.M., 43, 44, 45, 47, 57, 62, 72, 79, 99, 113, 116, 128, 144, 145
Barlow, W., 144
Barnes, M., 137
Bauer, G., 72
Bauer, H., 59
Beaumont, K., 139
Bernshtein, N., 37
Bernstein, N., 91
Berry, W.R., 147
Beukelman, D.R., 62, 147

Blonsky, E.R., 44, 57, 112
Booker, H.E., 144
Boshes, B., 44, 57, 112
Bosman, J., 13
Bouhuys, A., 11
Bratzlavsky, M., 71
Brodal, A., 54, 68, 72, 79
Brooks, V., 89
Brown, J., 34, 39, 41, 42, 44, 46, 58, 68, 69, 70, 72, 92, 108, 109
Brown, J.R., 56, 57, 71, 72, 79, 124, 126
Burke, R., 38, 97
Burns, M.O., 145

Caird, F., 123
Caligiuri, M. P., 147
Canter, G.J., 56
Cappa, S., 72
Capute, A., 10, 13, 93
Cariski, D., 79
Castellanos, F.X., 8
Celesia, G.G., 44, 45, 77, 112, 118, 120, 127, 128
Chadwick, D., 79
Chait, D., 135
Cleeland, C.S., 145
Cole, K., 36, 37, 43, 62, 64, 65, 89, 90, 91, 95, 105
Coleman, P.J., 144
Collins, M.J., 77, 118, 120, 128, 139
Cooper, I., 78, 137
Coyle, J., 60, 61, 78

Cramon, D. von, 73
Crickmay, M., 21, 74
Croft, C.B., 137
Culbertson, J., 10

Daniel, B., 45, 47, 57, 71, 79, 112,
    118, 120, 123, 127, 128, 129,
    134, 140, 144
D'Antonio, L., 135
Darley, F.L., 34, 39, 41, 42, 44,
    46, 56, 57, 71, 72, 79, 108, 109,
    124, 126
DeClerk, J., 15, 37, 91
Dedo, H., 136
DePaul, R., 145
Derouesne, J., 70
DeSanto, L.W., 136
Desmedt, J., 15, 36, 38, 40
Dickson, D., 137
Dickson, W., 137
Dietz, 114
Dubner, R., 39, 98
DuBois, A., 140
Dworkin, J.P., 144

Eecken, H. vander, 71
Ekbom, K., 23
Ender, P., 145
Evarts, E., 36, 64

Fairbanks, G., 146
Farrage, J., 118, 120, 138, 145
Fawcus, R., 21, 74
Ferguson, C., 1
Ferrendelli, J., 61
Ferry, P., 10
Feuer, E., 136
Finger, S., 54, 68, 75
Finley, W., 145
Fisher, H.B., 44, 57, 112
Fisher, M., 45
Fitzgibbons, P., 10
Fletcher, S., 17
Fra, L., 111
Freund, H.-J., 114
Fritzell, B., 37, 136, 137
Fromm, D., 37, 68

Fry, D., 96
Furr, M., 139

Gallistel, C., 36
Gandiglio, G., 111
Garnica, O., 2
Gay, T., 8, 38
Gazzaniga, M., 18
Gerstenbrand, F., 72
Gilbert, J., 20
Gilman, S., 43
Glaser, E., 137
Glaser, G., 43
Godaux, E., 38, 40
Goldberg, L., 97
Goldstein, K., 70
Gonzalez, J.B., 128
Goshan, E.L., 147
Gracco, K., 139
Gracco, V.L., 64
Granit, R., 35, 37, 40, 47
Greene, M.C.L., 132
Griggs, R., 72
Grillner, S., 36, 62, 64, 94, 95,
    96, 97
Grimby, L., 42, 43, 45
Grimm, R., 47
Guitar, B., 144
Gurfinkel, V., 37, 91

Haglund, S., 136
Hallen, O., 136
Hallett, M., 79
Hannerz, J., 42, 43, 45, 47
Hammarberg, R., 63
Hand, C.R., 145
Hanson, R., 47
Hanson, W.R., 115, 147
Hardy, J., 7, 21, 36, 37, 56, 65, 91,
    98, 99, 108, 140, 141
Harris, F., 68
Harris, R., 79
Harryman, S., 10, 13
Hartman, D.E., 144
Hassler, R., 93
Hassul, M., 8
Hecox, K., 15

Helm, N., 147
Hengl, W., 72
Hirano, M., 135
Hixon, T.J., 21, 36, 89, 98, 99,
    130, 131, 132, 134
Hoefer, P., 110
Honjow, I., 140
Honch, G., 72
Houk, J., 91
Hufschmidt, H., 110
Humphrey, T., 11
Hunker, C., 44, 45, 57, 62, 79, 99,
    112, 113, 114, 128

Ireland, E., 145
Isshiki, N., 140
Izdebski, K., 136

Jacobson, M., 11, 18
Jankovic, J., 71
Jarcho, L., 45, 46, 115
Jernelius, M., 23
Johns, D., 140, 141
Johnson, W., 106
Johnston, M., 60
Jurgens, U., 58

Kadanoff, D., 111
Kelso, J., 96
Kennedy, J., 57, 64
Kent, R.D., 4, 5, 8, 14, 16, 19, 37,
    38, 42, 57, 58, 59, 68, 90, 95,
    97, 142
Kinesbourne, M., 37
Knutsson, E., 136
Kornhuber, H., 35, 36, 43
Krival, M., 110
Kuehn, D., 37, 137
Kugelberg, E., 23

Ladefoged, P., 8, 15, 19, 37, 91
Langlois, A., 13
LaPointe, L., 47, 57, 62, 99, 118,
    126, 133, 146, 147
Larson, C., 34
LaVelle, W.E., 140
Leanderson, R., 45, 110

Lecours, A., 11, 12, 15, 18, 19,
    22, 70
Lee, R., 42, 45
Lenneberg, E., 56, 77, 142
Lennerstrand, G., 38, 39
Levik, Y.S., 37, 91
Lewin, M., 137
Lhermitte, F., 70
Lind, J., 13
Lindau, M., 15, 37, 91
Lindblom, B., 8, 38
Lindeman, R., 34
Linebaugh, C., 78, 118, 128
Logemann, J.A., 44, 57, 112
Lotz, W.K., 99, 119, 133, 135,
    139, 140
Lubker, J.F., 8, 37, 38, 62
Luria, A.R., 55, 58, 59, 94, 146
Luschei, E., 97
Lybolt, J., 118, 120, 138, 145

MacLean, P., 58, 92
MacNamara, R., 118
MacNeilage, P., 8, 15, 19, 37, 47,
    91, 97
Marquardt, T., 45, 111
Mateer, C., 94
Mateer, K., 36, 93
McCall, G., 137, 139
McClean, M., 23
McCusker, E., 72
McWilliams, B., 137
Meader, C., 56, 65, 70, 74
Metter, E.J., 115, 147
Metter, J.E., 124, 126
Meyerson, B., 45, 110
Miller, J., 25, 26, 98
Milner, E., 11, 13, 15, 18, 19, 22
Milner-Brown, H., 42, 45
Minifie, F., 29, 95, 97
Moll, K., 4, 38, 90
Moore, J., 58, 67, 68
Morimoto, M., 140
Morris, H., 141
Morris, S., 17, 25, 81
Mortimer, J., 45
Mountcastle, V., 66, 93

Moyers, R., 13, 16, 17
Muller, E., 8
Müller, E., 57
Murray, A., 59
Murry, T., 147
Muyskens, J., 55, 56, 65, 70, 74
Mysak, E., 58, 67, 68, 69, 71, 92, 99, 100

Nakazima, S., 14, 16
Nashner, L., 47
Nathanson, S., 13
Nelson, W., 63
Netsell, R., 4, 5, 6, 8, 23, 25, 26, 37, 38, 42, 43, 44, 45, 47, 57, 65, 67, 71, 79, 89, 90, 93, 98, 99, 105, 108, 112, 118, 119, 120, 123, 124, 125, 126, 127, 128, 129, 131, 132, 133, 134, 135, 138, 139, 140, 141, 142, 143, 144, 145
Netzky, M., 10
Niman, C., 145

Ohala, J., 20
Ojemann, G., 36, 94
Oller, K., 14, 17, 59

Paillard, J., 48
Palmer, F., 93
Papcun, G., 15, 37, 71, 91
Pellissier, J., 38, 39
Penfield, W., 68, 69
Perkell, J., 63
Persson, A., 36, 45, 110
Petajan, J., 45, 46, 115
Peterson, G., 28, 66
Ploog, D., 34, 35, 58, 68
Porter, R., 8
Pribam, K., 54
Prugger, M., 72
Purves, B., 20
Putnam, A.H.B., 130, 131
Putnam, T., 110

Quaglieri, C., 44

Rack, P., 95, 97
Rakoff, S.J., 137
Raleigh, M., 34, 35
Rieber, R., 56
Roberts, L., 68, 69
Robinson, B., 34, 35
Robinson, I., 71
Rosenbek, J.C., 47, 57, 61, 62, 77, 99, 105, 106, 118, 120, 126, 128, 133, 139, 146, 147
Rosenberg, R., 62
Rosin, P., 25, 26
Rubenstein, J., 10, 13
Rubow, R.T., 47, 57, 77, 115, 118, 120, 128, 132, 135, 139, 144
Rudick, R., 72
Rumpl, E., 72
Rutherford, D., 7, 65

Salyer, K., 140, 141
Schaltenbrand, G., 110
Scheibel, A., 11, 22, 36
Scheibel, M., 11, 22
Schneider, P., 110
Schriatzki, H., 136
Schweiger, J., 140, 141
Scott, A., 42
Scott, S., 123
Seif, M., 118, 120, 129
Serratrice, G., 38, 39
Sessle, B., 39, 93, 98
Shaughnessy, A., 99, 118, 133
Shelton, R., 139
Shipp, T., 136
Shirley, M., 17
Shohara, H., 55, 74
Shoup, J., 28, 66
Shprintzen, R.J., 137, 139
Skolnick, M., 137, 139
Sloan, R., 11
Smith, A., 47
Smitheran, J., 98, 134
Sommerfeld, R., 140
Standley, J., 145
Stark, R., 13
Stein, D., 54, 68, 75
Stein, R., 42

Steklis, H., 34, 35
Stetson, R., 56
Storey, A., 39, 98
Studdert-Kennedy, M., 33, 35
Sundberg, J., 136
Sussman, H., 47
Sutton, D., 34
Swift, E., 115, 132, 135

Tatton, W., 45
Terzuolo, C., 43
Thach, B., 14
Tinbergen, N., 54, 59
Trier, W., 139
Truby, H., 13
Tsukahara, N., 35

Vignolo, L., 72
Vignon, C., 38, 39
Vining, E., 10, 13
Viviani, P., 43
Vogel, M., 72

Wachtel, R., 93
Wall, P.D., 75
Wansley, R.A., 145

Ward, A., 94
Warren, D., 140
Warwick, R., 71
Watkin, K., 37
Watson, B., 132
Webster, D., 45
Weiffenbach, J., 14
Weiner, W., 45
Weismer, G., 79
Wertz, R.T., 146
Whitaker, H., 11, 22
White, N., 37
Whiting, H., 101
Wilder, C., 13
Williams, P., 71
Wolff, P., 13, 14, 37, 47, 54,
    59, 91
Woodruff, D., 13, 15

Yakovlev, P., 8, 9, 11, 15, 18, 19,
    21, 22
Yorkston, K.M., 62, 147

Zev Rymer, W., 91
Zimmerman, G., 47

SUBJECT INDEX

Page numbers in *italics* refer to
illustrations.

Adaptive control, and speech
    motor skill, 91
Adults, speech motor control in,
    2–7
Aerodynamic variables, in speech
    production, 3, *3*
Afferent influences, in speech
    motor control, 7, *7,* 64, *65*
  role of in speech, 94
Age, speech motor, 25, *26*
Ataxia, dysarthria, 42

Biofeedback, 129, 130. See also
    Instrumental methods, for
    treating dysarthria.
"Babbler" stage (3 to 12 months),
    14–17
  development of motor control in,
    16
  neural maturation in, 15
Behavioral methods, for treating
    dysarthria, 126, 129
  for all components
    simultaneously, 146
  laryngeal system, 134
  orofacial system, 141
  respiratory system, 131
  velopharyngeal system, 138
Bite–block, for treating dysarthria,
    145

Brain injury, recovery from, 75
Broca's area, as final motor
    pathway for speech, 36
Brodal, experiences of following
    stroke, 79–81

Cerebellum, as velocity adjustor of
    muscle contractions, 44
  disorders of, and dysarthria, 42
Clinician, speech, as researcher,
    105
Clinician, speech, Johnson's three
    questions for, 106
Cognition, role of neuro-
    transmitters and, 60
Communication disorders,
    interactionist model of, 55
Contrastive stress drill, for treating
    dysarthria, 145
"Critical" periods, of maturation,
    10

Delayed auditory feedback, for
    treating dysarthria, 147
Dendrites, growth of, 22
Differentiation, embryonic, 21
Distributed systems and functions,
    in speech motor control, 66,
    93
Dysarthria(s), as speech motor
    control problem, 107
  cerebellar disorders and, 42
  classification of, 40–47
  definition of, 53

developmental, 47
documentation and reevaluation
    of treatment, 119
flaccid, 41
forms of, 41–47, 109
historical developments of
    neurobiologic view, 55
hypertonia of lips in, 111, 113
nervous system and, 57. See also
    Nervous system.
neuropathology and, 67–75
neurobiologic view of, 53–83
orofacial tremor in, 114
Parkinson's disease and, 44
peripheral nervous system
    lesions and, 41
physiologic approach to, 47
physiologic evaluation of, 125
physiological studies of,
    108–116
  current developments,
      110–115
  Hunker and Abbs, 114
  Hunker et al., 113
  Leandersson et al., 110
  Marquardt, 111
  Mayo Clinic study, 109
perceptual physiologic studies
    of, 108, 109
  Netsell et al., 112
  relevance to treatment,
      116–119
selecting and sequencing
    treatment goals, 118
severity of impairment in, 127
speech mechanism examination
    in, 117, *117*
speech motor control and,
    61–66. See also *Speech
    motor control.*
speech patterns in, physiologic
    interpretation of, 116
speech therapy and, 81
theoretical issues affecting
    treatment, 98
treatment of, 76–82, 123–148
  age of patient and, 77

automatic adjustments by
    patient and, 77
behavioral methods, 126, 129
  for all functional compo-
      nents simultaneously, 146
  for laryngeal component,
      133–137
  for orofacial component,
      141
  for respiratory component,
      131
  for velopharyngeal compo-
      nent, 138
documenting speech changes
    and, 79
effects of, 77, 78
factors influencing, 76, 126,
    129
for all functional components
    simultaneously, 146–148
implications of theoretical
    issues, 100
instrumental methods, 126,
    129
instrumental, for all functional
    components simultaneously,
    147
  for laryngeal component,
      134
  for orofacial component,
      144
  for respiratory component,
      132
  for velopharyngeal compo-
      nent, 139
methods of, 79, 126, 129,
    130–148
neurologic status of patient
    and, 76
neurophysiologic approach,
    79
passive and skilled movements
    and, 80
pathophysiology and, 127
patient's communication needs
    and, 130
patient's history and, 76

patient's medical status and, 128

patient's support systems and, 78

personality and intelligence of patient and, 78

physiological approach to, 107, 116–119, 124–130

prosthetic methods, 126, 129

  for laryngeal component, 135

  for orofacial component, 145

  for respiratory component, 133

  for velopharyngeal component, 139

shared versus specialized mechanisms for, 74, 81

time available for, 129

vegetative, 21

unanswered questions about, 119

Dysphonia, spastic, recurrent laryngeal nerve resection for, 136

Efferent processes, in speech motor control, 7, *7*, 65, *65*

Electrolarynx, 137

Electromyography, in treating orofacial components of dysarthria, 144

Embryonic differentiation, 21

Ethology, and speech motor control, 34

Facilitation, in speech production, 143

Feedback, in speech motor control, 64, *64*, 95

Feedforward, in speech motor control, 64, *64*, 95

Flaccid dysarthria, 41

Flap, pharyngeal, in treating dysarthria, 140

Force ramp, of muscles, 40

Functional components, of speech mechanism, 2, *3*

Gestural reorganization, for treating dysarthria, 145

Hypertonia, of lip muscles, in dysarthria, 111, 113

Injury, brain, recovery from, 75

Instrumental methods, for treating dysarthria, 125, 126, 129

  for all components simultaneously, 147

  laryngeal system, 134

  orofacial system, 144

  respiratory system, 132

  velopharyngeal system, 139

Jaw sling, for treating dysarthria, 145

Language development, myelination and, *12*

Laryngeal nerve, recurrent, resection of, 136

  in treatment of dysarthrias, 133–137

Laryngeal system, as functional component of speech, 125, *125*, 133–137

Limbic system, neuropathology and, 68

Lips, feedback and feedforward movements, 64, *64*

  hypertonia of, in dysarthria, 111, 113

"Locked-in" syndrome, 72

Maturation, nervous system. See *Nervous system, maturation of.*

Metrics, of normal speech, 90

Motor acts, afferent construction of, 94

Motor control, development of, in "babbler" stage, 16

in neonatal period, 13
in prenatal period, 11
in toddler stage, 18
in refinement period, 20
of speech. See *Speech motor
    control*.
Motor equivalence, speech, *62,* 63
Movements, lip, feedback and
    feedforward mechanisms,
    64, *64*
  for syllables [apa], *62*
  passive and skilled, in recovery
    from stroke, 80
  speech, nature of, 23
    neural origins of, 20
    reflexive, 23, *24*
  upper airway, for [i] vowel,
    63, *63*
  vegetative, embryonic develop-
    ment of, 21
    nature of, 23
  vocal tract, for speech, 142, 143
    speech versus nonspeech acts
    and, 98
Muscle action potentials, from
    orbicularis oris muscle for
    /p/ and /b/, *41*
Muscle forcing functions, in
    speech, 40
  disorders of, 40
Myelination, and speech and
    language development, *12*
  in "babbler" stage, *12,* 15
  in neonatal period, 12, *12*
  in prenatal period, 11, *12*
  in refinement period, *12,* 19
  in toddler stage, *12,* 18
  of nervous system, 22

Neocortical system, neuropathol-
    ogy and, 68
Neonatal period, development of
    motor control in, 13
  neural maturation in 12, *12*
Nervous system. See also *Speech
    motor control*.
  and neural origins of speech

movements, 20–25
  anterior versus posterior systems
    in, 69–71
  continuum of actions and
    modes of control in, 95
  dendritic growth in, 22
  distributed functions and,
    71–73, 93
  dysarthria and, 57. See also
    Dysarthria.
  embryonic differentiation of, 21
  evolving and interactive systems
    in, 67–71
  "hard wiring" of, 18
  levels of command specificity in,
    95
  maturation of, and speech motor
    control, 8–20
    "babbler" stage (3 to 12
    months), 14
    criteria for, 9
    "critical" and "sensitive"
    periods of, 10
    neonatal period, 12–14
    prenatal period, 11
    refinement period, 19
    toddler period, 17–19
  myelination of, 11, *12,* 15, 18,
    19, 22
  ontogeny of, 59, 92
  pathology of, and dysarthria, 67
  phylogeny of, 57, 92
  recovery from brain injury and,
    75
  restricted lesions and, 71–73
  reticular, limbic, and neocortical
    systems in, 67
  shared versus specialized neur-
    onal mechanisms, 74, 81
Neural maturation. See *Nervous
    system, maturation of*.
Neurologic disorders, speech
    motor control and, 33–48
Neurotransmitters, role of, in
    nervous system, 60

Ontogeny, of nervous system, 59,

92
Orofacial system, as functional
    component of speech, 125,
    141–145
  in treatment of dysarthrias,
    141–145
Oscilloscope, in treating dysarthria,
    135

Pacing board, for treating dysar-
    thria, 147
Palatal lift prosthesis, for treating
    dysarthria, 139
Parkinson's disease, dysarthria
    and, 44, 109, 110–115
Peripheral dependencies, principle
    of, in treating dysarthrias,
    127
Peripheral nervous system, lesions
    of, and dysarthria, 41
Pharyngeal flap, in treating dysar-
    thria, 140
Phylogeny, of nervous system, 57,
    92
Physiological studies, of dysarthria
    (see Dysarthria, physiologi-
    cal studies of)
Precision, of normal speech, 91
Prenatal period, development of
    motor control in, 11
  neural maturation in, 11, 12
Prosthesis, palatal lift, for treating
    dysarthria, 139
Prosthestic methods, for treating
    dysarthrias, 126, 129
  laryngeal system, 135
  orofacial system, 145
  respiratory system, 133
  velopharyngeal system, 139

Refinement period, development of
    motor control in, 20
  neural maturation in, 19
Reflex circuits, for speech, 23, 24
Respiratory system, as functional
    component of speech, 125,
    125, 130–133

  in treatment of dysarthrias,
    130–133
Reticular system, neuropathology
    and, 67
Rhinomanometry, in treating
    dysarthria, 140

"Sensitive" periods, of maturation,
    10, 27
Somatoafference, role of in speech,
    94
Sound production, in infant, 14
Spastic dysphonia, recurrent
    laryngeal nerve resection
    for, 136
Spatial-temporal coordination, in
    speech motor control, 20,
    61, 62
Speech. See also Speech motor
    control; Speech production.
  acquisition of, 2–8
  adult models of, 2–7
  afferent processes, 64, 65, 94
  as motor control system, 8, 33
  as motor skill, 1, 27, 36
  continuum of actions and modes
    of control in, 97
  development of, and myelination,
    12
  functional components of, 124,
    125, 125
  learning to talk, 65, 65
  motor control of. See Speech
    motor control.
  motor equivalence and, 62, 63
  motor milestones of, 25, 26
  muscle contractile forces in, 38
  neural mechanisms of, evalu-
    ating, 92, 98
    speech versus nonspeech acts
      and, 98
    testing component function
      and adaptive control, 99
  normal, metrics of, 90
  precision capabilities of, 90
  rehabilitation of, force of inner-
    vation and, 81

shared versus specialized neuronal mechanisms for, 74, 81
spatial-temporal goals in, *61,* 62
Speech clinician, as clinical researcher, 105
  Johnson's three questions for, 106
Speech disorders, functional systems analysis of, 55
Speech mechanism, examination of, 117, *117*
  functional components of, 2, *3*
Speech, motor age, 25, *26*
Speech motor control. See also *Motor control, development of.*
  acquisition of, 1–28, *7,* 65, *65*
  adaptive control and, 91
  afferent influences in, 7, *7,* 64, *65*
  and nervous system maturation, 8–20
  development of gross coordinations in, 19
  disorders of, 39–48
  distributed systems in, 66
  dysarthria and, 107. See also *Dysarthria.*
  efferent processes in, 7, *7,* 65, *65*
  ethologic considerations, 34
  evaluation of dysarthrias and, 61–66
  evolutionary influences on, 34
  facilitating development of, 100
  feedback and feedforward in, 64, *64,* 95
  in adults, 3–7
  levels of command specificity in, 95
  motor equivalence in, *62,* 63
  neocortical system in, 35
  neural maturation and, 8–20
  neural pathways and muscles in, 34, *35, 67*

neurologic disorders and, 33–48
neuropathology and, 67–75
normal, 38
restoration of, 100
"sensitive" period in acquisition, 27
spatial-temporal coordination in, 20, 27, *61,* 62
speech motor age and, 25, *26*
theoretical issues with clinical impact, 89–102
Speech movements, neural origins of, 20
Speech production, aerodynamic variables in, *3.* See also *Speech.*
  differentiating movements in, 142
  exaggerating movements in, 143
  for *ea* and *m* sounds, *6*
  for vowel *i* (midsaggital drawings), *5*
  structures involved in, *3*

Teflon injections, for unilateral vocal fold paralysis, 136
Toddler period, development of motor control in, 18
  neural maturation in, 18
Treatment of dysarthria. See *Dysarthria.*
Tremor, orofacial, in dysarthria, 114

Vegetative therapy, for speech disorders, 21
Velopharyngeal system, as functional component of speech, 125, *125,* 137–141
  in treating dysarthrias, 137–141
Videofiberoptics, for treating dysarthria, 135
Voice amplifier, portable, 132
Voice light, in treating dysarthria, 135

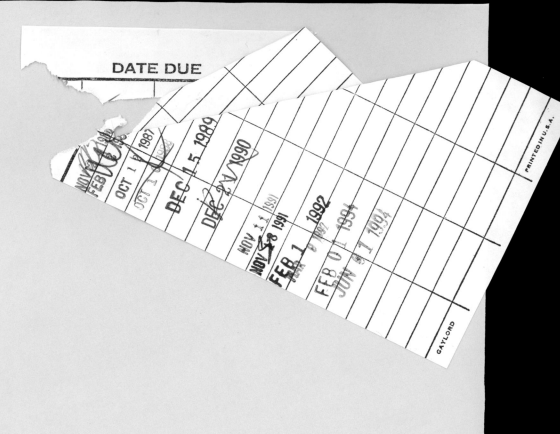